MAXIMIZE YOUR TESTOSTERONE AT ANY AGE!

Improve

- erections
- muscular size and strength
- energy level
- mood
- heart health
- longevity
- prostate health
- bone health
- and much more!

J.M. SWARTZ M.D.
Y.L. WRIGHT M.A.

Published and distributed worldwide by:
LULU PRESS, INC., 627 Davis Drive, Morrisville, NC 27560

Printed in the United States of America

ISBN: 978-0-359-58775-9

MEDICAL DISCLAIMER:

The following text contains the opinions and ideas of the authors. Careful attention has been paid to insure the accuracy of the information, but the authors and the publisher cannot assume responsibility for the validity or consequences of its use. This information is not intended to diagnose or treat any disease. We are only providing education and our point of view. The authors are not rendering medical, health, or any other professional services. See your medical or health professional concerning any health concerns or before following any suggestions made in this book or drawing inferences from it. The authors specifically disclaim all responsibility for any liability, loss, or risk incurred as a direct or indirect consequence of using this book's contents. Any use of the information found in this book is the sole responsibility of the reader. Any suggestions found in this book are to be followed only under the supervision of a medical doctor and/or a trained dentist. The authors have no financial ties to any products discussed in this book.

DEDICATION: "MAXIMIZE YOUR TESTOSTERONE AT ANY AGE!" was written for you. If even one person finds their way out of chronic disease and suffering into health, it has been worth it.

THIS IS BOOK 9 IN THE "BIOIDENTICAL HORMONES" BOOK SERIES. These books may be read separately or as a series.

Read this book and learn how to raise your testosterone levels into the optimum range for fantastic health, no matter how young or how old you are. Read the stories of men of all ages who came in to Dr. Joe's office with interesting hormonal challenges that had baffled other doctors. Learn how their problems were untangled, diagnosed, and successfully treated, despite previously not getting help from one or more traditional physicians.

Using prescription testosterone causes infertility and shrinking testicles. Read the stories of two men who were able to bring their testosterone up AND maintain fertility WITHOUT using prescription testosterone. Other stories are about men who needed to balance other hormones before their testosterone could go up.

OTHER BOOKS BY J.M. SWARTZ, M.D. AND Y.L. WRIGHT, M.A.:

"MEN'S HORMONES MADE EASY! How to Treat: Low Testosterone, Low Growth Hormone, Erectile Dysfunction, BPH, Andropause, Insulin Resistance, Adrenal Fatigue, Thyroid, Osteoporosis, High Estrogen, and DHT!" Prevent and Reverse: Manopause, Prostate Issues, Heart Disease, and Cancer. See how hormone issues at any age may: Wreck your relationship. Make you fat. Accelerate aging and death. Learn how to SAFELY: Improve your sexual performance. Increase your energy, motivation, and sex drive. Strengthen muscles and bones. This book is designed to be a workbook in anti-aging medicine for self-responsible men who want to intelligently work with their physicians for optimal life and longevity. It is also an update on the diagnosis and treatment of mild, moderate, and severe hormonal problems for physicians who have been unable to keep up-to-date on anti-aging medicine.

"BIOIDENTICAL HORMONES MADE EASY!" Learn about bioidentical hormone replacement therapy (BHRT) for women in a quick and easy book.

"SECRETS ABOUT GROWTH HORMONE TO BUILD MUSCLE, INCREASE BONE DENSITY, AND BURN BODY FAT!" See how Growth Hormone levels drop as we get older, when to intervene, and what treatment options are available to optimize health.

"SECRETS ABOUT BIOIDENTICAL HORMONES to Lose Fat and Prevent Cancer, Heart Disease, Menopause, and Andropause by Optimizing Adrenals, Thyroid, Estrogen, Progesterone, Testosterone, and Growth Hormone!" Learn about the leading edge of anti-aging medicine--Bioidentical Hormone Therapy. Discover how to diagnose hormonal abnormalities. You will also be given treatment options.   Learn how hormones become unbalanced, especially during menopause and andropause.

"FAT LOSS SECRETS THAT REALLY WORK:Balance Your Hormones: Insulin, Estrogen, Progesterone, Testosterone, Thyroid, Cortisol, and DHEA!" Find out exactly how to correct the hormonal problems that prevent you from losing fat, especially belly fat, and how to normalize your weight for the rest of your life.

"SECRETS ABOUT THE HCG DIET! Treatment Guide, Controversy, Benefits, Risks, Side Effects, and Contraindications." Discover the answers to: What is hCG? How does hCG work? How is it used in a program to lose weight?

"SECRETS to LOSE TOXIC BELLY FAT! Heal Your Sick Metabolism Using State-Of-The-Art Medical Testing and Treatment With Detoxification, Diet, Lifestyle, Supplements, and Bioidentical Hormones." Toxic belly fat is a parasite that preserves itself at the expense of its host -- YOU! Lose toxic belly fat and regain metabolic health by correcting the sick metabolism associated with toxic belly fat.

"THE WISDOM OF BIOIDENTICAL HORMONES In Menopause, Perimenopause, and Premenopause! Unleash the power of Estrogen,

Progesterone, Testosterone, Cortisol, DHEA, Growth Hormone, Pregnenolone, Oxytocin, Vitamin D3, and Melatonin!" THE WISDOM OF BIOIDENTICAL HORMONES lies in knowing when and how to use them. This book can help you determine which methods of bioidentical hormone replacement therapy (BHRT), if any, may work best for YOU, no matter how old you are, whether you are in menopause, perimenopause, or even younger. To really feel at your best, you may or may not need bioidentical hormone replacement. Are bioidentical hormones safe?   Do they cause cancer? Are there side effects? When should you begin to use them? What tests are needed? How can you find a doctor who will prescribe the bioidentical hormones that will work best for you? Get this book and learn the answers to all of these questions.

"TOXIC TEETH: How a Biological (Holistic) Dentist Can Help You Cure Cancer, Facial Pain, Autoimmune, Heart, and Other Disease Caused By Infected Gums, Root Canals, Jawbone Cavitations, and Toxic Metals." TOXIC TEETH will help you to understand exactly what options you really do have about your dentistry and your health.   What exactly are the consequences of those common dental procedures your dentist is performing on you and your family?   Is it possible that the most common dental procedures practiced by nearly all dentists put you at a high risk for life-threatening illness? Read TOXIC TEETH to see how you can easily prevent problems with your teeth and gums before they ever happen and reverse problems that you may already be experiencing.

"KETO SMART!: Heal Your Brain and Body With the Ten-Step Action Plan Scientifically Proven to Prevent or Reverse Obesity, Memory Loss, Alzheimer's, Diabetes, Autoimmunity, Cancer, and Heart Disease."   The KETO SMART 10-step protocol is MUCH more than just following a ketogenic diet. The KETO SMART 10-step protocol is a comprehensive program of self-healing. Follow the KETO SMART ten easy action steps, and soon your thinking mind will become as penetrating as the depths of a pristine alpine lake on a quiet sunny morning.

CONTENTS

CHAPTER 1. THINKING OUTSIDE THE BOX.

This book was written by Joe Swartz, M.D. and Yvonne Wright, M.A. We are a husband and wife team with a mission to enlighten people about how to optimize their hormones. That's why we have written the "Bioidentical Hormones" book series.

Dr. Joe is a family-practice physician who specializes in very difficult problems. His patients arrive with puzzling problems that have not been successfully treated by any other practitioners. Yvonne is the office and family manager, book writer, and editor. People come to Dr. Joe's office when they are not happy with the medical advice and treatment that they have been getting from physicians who practice the traditional standard-of-care medicine.

Dr. Joe is not afraid to think outside the box. He likes to get to the bottom of things and find out what is really causing a person's problems.

That's the kind of thinking that is needed to optimize hormones. Hormones can be tricky. You have to be a detective and figure out what is causing what.

You can't just give a prescription to your patient after talking to him for ten minutes and expect all of his problems to disappear. You need to listen to his story, ask the right questions, do the right tests, and then develop a thoughtful diagnosis and a comprehensive treatment plan.

This book includes the stories of men who came to Dr. Joe's office with all kinds of interesting hormonal challenges that had baffled other doctors. We will discuss how their problems were untangled, deciphered, diagnosed, and successfully treated, despite not being able to get help from one or more traditional physicians.

Their stories may seem unusual, but are, in fact, common examples of the complex interactions that are often seen with hormones and other medical problems. Perhaps you will be able to personally relate to some of the hormone situations that we will discuss. Or you may know of someone who might benefit from the wisdom that we will share in these pages. In any event, we hope that you enjoy learning how a medical sleuth gets to the bottom of these men's hormone imbalances, bringing their testosterone levels up into the optimal ranges, often without the need for prescription testosterone treatments.

Traditional doctors comply with standard-of-care.

The type of doctor that you choose to see is extremely important when it comes down to whether or not you are going to get help to bring your hormones into balance.

The traditional medical establishment follows rules that may not be in your best interests, especially when it comes to hormone treatments. Most of my patients have previously seen one or more conventional physicians who have refused to treat their hormonal problems, because their laboratory test results did not fit into conventional medicine's standard-of-care strict criteria for hormonal imbalance.

When you consult a traditional medical doctor, you may be allowing yourself to be set-up for continuing health deterioration. You may have to wait until your hormone problems become so severe that your lab results finally look bad enough to get a prescription. That could be five years or ten years or twenty years from now. All the while your health continues to get worse.

The most dangerous situation is where hormone imbalances are not recognized and symptoms are treated with pharmaceutical drugs. Conventionally-educated doctors have not been trained to recognize hormone imbalances. Instead, they pull out their prescription pad to treat the symptoms of disease. They have not been trained to look for the causes of disease.

Anti-aging medicine for optimal hormonal health.

Anti-aging doctors take a different approach to balancing hormones. The longer you persist in a state of hormonal imbalance, the worse things will become, so the anti-aging doctor is eager to treat mild and moderate hormonal dysfunction BEFORE it becomes severe.

I treat people with mild to moderate hormonal imbalances before the problems become severe. This is different from the conventional medicine approach of waiting until hormone problems deteriorate to the point of severity. As an anti-aging physician, trained by the American Academy of Anti-Aging Medicine (A4M), I believe that every man and woman has the right to receive treatment to optimize their hormones, no matter how severe the hormonal imbalance may be.

You will understand more about the differences between conventional medicine and anti-aging medicine as you listen to the stories of the men who have come to see me because they are concerned about their hormones.

All of the hormones work together.

As you read these men's stories, you will begin to realize that successful hormone treatment needs to follow a particular order. For instance, treating the thyroid without first addressing adrenal dysfunction may result in becoming even more tired and miserable. Or if growth hormone is sufficiently depressed, you can't fix the adrenals until that growth hormone deficiency is treated. And if testosterone is low due to a problem in the pituitary gland in the brain, you have to address that problem first.

We need to evaluate all of the hormones before we can arrive at a diagnosis and treatment plan that works. You have to look at all of the hormones in order to develop a game plan that works. Otherwise you are just spinning your wheels or even going backward.

Weigh the risks against the benefits.

If you do decide to use testosterone therapy, learn how to do it safely. Learn about all of the risks, as well as the benefits. Learn about possible adverse effects and contraindications (conditions that would make testosterone therapy dangerous for you). Blood clots associated with testosterone treatment are currently generating class-action lawsuits. Other medical concerns about the true risk of testosterone therapy have also been raised.

Testosterone therapy shrinks your testicles and takes away your ability to father a child if you take it long enough. Read on to find out about alternative hormone treatments that may work to raise your testosterone without resulting in a loss of fertility and a decrease in testicular volume. All of the concerns must be weighed against potential benefits before jumping in and beginning treatment with testosterone.

Raising low testosterone in young men.

Low testosterone doesn't just happen to older men.[1] Young men may also have low levels of testosterone that have gone undetected. Although andropause typically affects men in their fifties and older, testosterone may begin to decline significantly even in men who are much younger.

Depending on the reason, hormonal loss in young men can often be reversed. It depends on the reason for the low testosterone. Young men may be able to bring their testosterone levels up with lifestyle,[2] diet, and supplements alone.

Correcting low T without lowering sperm count.

Low testosterone in younger men can often be corrected with prescription hormones without lowering sperm count, if the objective is to be able to father children. To demonstrate how this can be possible, listen now to the stories of two young men with similar hormone problems but coming from different causes. Both show symptoms of low testosterone and do not wish to lose their fertility. We will discuss their histories, tests, diagnoses, and treatments.

First let's listen to Ted's story of hormone dissatisfaction and see how we were able to help him and his wife to become happier. Then we will see how Sam was able to correct his symptoms of testosterone deficiency in an entirely different way.

CHAPTER 2. TED'S ONLY PROBLEM IS HIS WIFE.

TED IS 43 YEARS OLD. HE CAME TO SEE ME ONE DREARY, COLD JANUARY DAY BECAUSE HIS WIFE SENT HIM. Ted's mood matches the weather. He is not happy at all.

His chief complaint today is his wife. "I'm here because my wife is bitching at me. There's nothing wrong with me. SHE's the one with the problem." Ted's childless 38-year old wife, Cheryl, is running out of time. Cheryl desperately wants to get pregnant. Cheryl blames Ted for their inability to conceive.

Ted explains, "The duration and fullness of my erections are not the same as they used to be. But I can still get it up, Doc. I think it's just that her bitching at me all the time upsets me. That's my problem. I'm a healthy guy, but here I am."

The history screen gives us some clues.

I tell Ted, "Let's just talk a minute and do a quick history screen, especially looking at your hormones--thyroid, adrenals, and sex hormones. Let's see what may be concerning your wife."

Thyroid questions and answers.

"First, let's look at your thyroid. Have you been gaining or losing weight?"

"No, my weight has been stable."

"Do you tend to be constipated?"

"Not really, but my bowel movements are not that great."

"Are you cold when you would not expect yourself to be cold? Are you colder now than you were in the past?"

"No."

"Are you fatigued?"

"No."

"Have you or your wife noticed that your thinking is slower?"

"We have noticed that something is not quite on. I seem to be slower but don't really care."

Adrenal function is critical.

"Next, let's look at your adrenal function." How is your sleep?"

"My sleep is not restful any more. I sleep longer, but don't feel refreshed. I feel wired but tired."

"Do you find that you are easily affected by stress? How stressful do you rate your life—mild, moderate, or severe?"

"I work in sales. What do you think? It seems like there is never enough time in the day to get things done."

"Do you have any episodes of blood sugar instability? Do you ever have periods of low blood sugar where you feel shaky, hungry, and faint followed by accelerated heart rate?"

"I remember experiencing that in the past year occasionally."

From his symptoms, we can conclude that Ted's adrenals are unable to cope with the stress in his life. Testing will clarify the extent of the adrenal dysfunction.

All of the sex hormones need to be considered.

"Next, let's look at the sex hormones. Have you noticed a loss of muscle mass over the past year? Are you weaker than you would expect to be based upon your level of activity and how you were a year ago?"

"Yes. I have definitely noticed more weakness."

"You said that you don't have fatigue. But how would you rate your vital energy—resistance to infection, ability to stress yourself emotionally, physically. Do you hold up under stress?"

"It's not what it was a year ago. In fact, it's not been good for the past five years."

"How is your libido? This is not your ability to perform, but your pure interest in sex."

"It is definitely not what it was five years ago."

"As I understand it, you do not have erectile dysfunction—an inability to perform, but your vitality has also diminished over the past five years."

"That would be an accurate statement."

Low testosterone is suspected.

Further questioning revealed that Ted had many symptoms of low testosterone:

- He no longer had morning erections.
- His interest in sex had diminished.
- He was depressed.
- His muscle mass was lower than it was a few years ago despite working out with weights. He didn't feel the increased strength and muscle growth that weight lifting had given him in the past.
- His sexual function was "OK," but it took more stimulation to arouse him.
- He had shorter duration of erections with less volume of ejaculate.

High DHT causes issues.

I explain to Ted, "Besides the common sex hormone problem of low testosterone, another important sex hormone (called DHT) can cause issues when it gets too high."

"Have you had any increased hair loss, especially male pattern baldness?"

"No."

"Have you had any prostate symptoms—decreased stream of urine, post-void dribbling, getting up at night more frequently to urinate?"

"No."

"Have you had a PSA in the past year?"

"No."

"We'll get one."

Estrogen is too high in many men.

I tell Ted, **"For many men, the female hormone, estrogen, may be too high."**

"Have you noticed any increased fat tissue in your breast area?"

"Yes, a bit fuller in the breasts."

"Has your belly fat increased?"

"Yes, despite doing more ab work."

"Do you feel like you are more passive in your relationship with your wife than you were a year or more ago?"

"I am sure that I have not been passive, but I have to admit that my vitality has been more limited for everything."

Testing clarifies Ted's hormone issues.

I do a physical exam and everything appears normal. I recommend some blood tests.

Some blood tests are considered essential, others ideal. The decision about which tests to get is how much of a financial burden it will be. All of these tests will have to paid for out of pocket.

Insurance won't pay for blood tests on a healthy-appearing guy. I explain to Ted that if he doesn't want to pay for the tests now, he could just wait until he gets sick enough to the point where insurance will pay for the tests. But that could be five or ten years from now. "If you do have hormonal deficiency now that is causing your problems, your health will permanently deteriorate until these deficiencies are corrected.

My advice is that health is worth more than gold. The wise path is the middle way—to get the essential testing and then follow up with the tests that are most appropriate and beneficial.

I recommend as essential—a total and free testosterone, an LH, and an IGF-1 to screen for growth hormone deficiency. I would also like to get four-point cortisol testing for the adrenals and a TSH as a screen for thyroid. It's good to get all these done now."

"OK, doc."

"I will the order the tests."

Ted's testosterone levels were below normal. His blood test revealed that Ted's testosterone levels were below normal. I emphasize the point that, "If you ever start using testosterone, you will become progressively infertile." Since fertility is his wife's main concern, testosterone supplementation at this point would be counterproductive to his relationship.

Instead of just immediately throwing testosterone prescriptions at Ted, we looked for the reasons why his testosterone was low. Maybe we could bring his testosterone up some other way, without the negative side effects that come with testosterone supplementation.

When working normally, a gland in the brain, called the pituitary gland, secretes enough hormones to kick the testes into gear to make enough testosterone. The hormone that prods the testes into action to produce testosterone is called LH (luteinizing hormone).

Ted's LH was way too low. Without enough LH, his testes could not make enough testosterone to keep him healthy. This means that the problem was probably not in the testes, but was definitely in the brain, because the pituitary gland (the master controller of the body) was not working properly.

Diagnosis: Low LH hypogonadism.

LH testing showed us that the low testosterone problem was caused in Ted's brain, not in his testes, where the testosterone is produced.

His diagnosis was low LH hypogonadism. He was severely deficient in testosterone and his pituitary was doing nothing to stimulate the testes to produce more testosterone. Ted's depression, low sex drive, and loss of muscle mass were the result of insufficient hormones secreted from his brain! We would have to explore ways to raise Ted's LH. If we could raise his LH, his testosterone would probably come up, as well.

Why is Ted's pituitary not working right?

Next we needed to find out why his pituitary was not functioning properly.

- High on our list of probabilities would be heavy metal toxicity, especially mercury.

- The next consideration would be inflammatory diseases that could be affecting the pituitary.

- Closely related, but a separate issue, would be to rule out leaky gut.

- Autoimmune disorders must be excluded.

- There was no real indication that we should consider infectious disease.

- A teeny tumor of the pituitary is high on the list of traditional doctors, but because low LH hypogonadism is now such a frequent disease, this possibility rates very low. Evaluation for this possibility by traditional medicine involves some invasive technology that is best avoided if possible.

- If all of these turn out to be negative, we may be looking at a toxin that we can't identify. There are markers like how oxidized are the walls of your cells that would indicate a mysterious injurious toxin.

I recommended the following tests: A chelated heavy metal screen and comprehensive mercury studies testing for multiple inflammatory markers.

Healing the sick adrenals is the first concern.

The first thing that Ted needed to do was to heal his sick adrenals. Testing showed us that the daily rhythm of secretion of cortisol, an adrenal hormone, was out of whack. Without a proper rhythm of stress hormones coming from the adrenals, his other hormones could never work well. Just healing the adrenals would allow all of his other hormones to work better. I instructed Ted to follow these five steps to heal his sick adrenals.

Ted needed to change his diet.

(1) Ted had to drastically changing his eating habits. Ted had to stop eating dead things and eat only live foods. Foods that are processed or canned are dead with no life vitality left in them. Ted needed to learn that in a typical large grocery store, 80% of the products in the store were now unavailable to him, mainly because they are processed and filled with chemicals.

To be serious about his health, Ted also had to avoid all high-glycemic carbohydrates (foods that spike blood sugar). From now on, if Ted ate any carbohydrate he always had to buffer it with fat and protein. He could have a half of a potato, but he had to put butter or sour cream on it. He had to have 40% of his diet in high quality fats to give his body plenty of good fats and cholesterol every day. These good fats would help him to build up levels of testosterone. He needed to eat protein at every meal.

If he began to eat this way, he wouldn't make excessive amounts of cholesterol in his liver. I explained to Ted that stroke and heart attack from hardening of the arteries are inflammatory diseases caused by smoking, diabetes, and toxicity. These diseases are not caused just by eating healthy foods with cholesterol in them.

I explained that we were giving him the building blocks for health. I warned Ted that he would initially gain weight, but after he healed his sick metabolism, he would be able to lose the weight. We had to stop the high sugar levels that were coating every cell in his body with sugar.

Daily exercise is a must.

(2) He needs to begin to exercise daily, not missing a day, with moderate activity, avoiding over-exercising. He needs to get up and go to the gym in the morning before work, whether he feels like it or not. He needs to hire a personal trainer to kick his rear end into gear. Paying a personal trainer will hold him accountable to show up and work out hard every day and motivate Ted to take responsibility for his health.

At the same time, Ted needs to stop exercising before he feels completely exhausted. He should walk out of the gym feeling like he still has enough energy to do the whole work-out again.

Without diet and exercise, it is impossible to regain health. You can take all of the pills in the world, but you will not get health from them. You can do everything else right, but if you do not eat right and exercise, you will not be successful.

Ted needs to take adaptogens.

(3) In addition to changing his diet and exercising, Ted also needs to start taking adaptogens. Adaptogens are herbs that would not only help heal his adrenals but would also heal his brain and his heart, vital organs that are damaged by adrenal dysfunction. Ashwagandha is the most important adaptogen to heal the adrenals.

Sleep is critical.

(4) The next most important change to make is for Ted to get plenty of deep, restorative sleep. He must normalize his sleep patterns and practice good sleep hygiene. He needs to begin winding down at 9 PM, avoiding anything that would activate him, like TV or even exercise. An hour before bedtime, he should take phosphatidylserine, a food-grade supplement made from lecithin. This brings down levels of stress hormones, allowing deeper sleep. He is to be in bed by 10 pm, relaxing and/or meditating.

Ted must stop doing and bring being into his life.

(5) Ted must avoid type-A behavior (doing-doing-doing and time-urgent behavior) and bring more "being" into his life. Taking time to enjoy meals, meditation, and yoga are great ways to do this.

Bringing up Ted's low testosterone.

After implementing the lifestyle changes to heal his adrenals, the next thing for Ted to do was to raise his testosterone. Ted's testosterone was seriously low. Although some young men can raise low testosterone simply by using herbal supplements and losing weight with dietary changes and exercise, Ted was way beyond the point for those strategies to work effectively. We would have to look at other options.

We had determined that Ted's low testosterone was caused by low secretion of hormones in his brain. (This is not the case with all men, but it was in Ted's case.) Ted's brain wasn't secreting enough luteinizing hormone (LH) to stimulate his testes to produce enough testosterone.

Because of his young age, Ted had two choices to raise his testosterone:

(1) To use hCG (human Chorionic Gonadotropin) (which acts like LH) to stimulate his own testes to produce more testosterone. HCG usually works to raise testosterone only for about three years. If we could not find a way to heal the problem in the brain within those three years, testosterone replacement would then be necessary.

(2) Just give him supplemental bioidentical testosterone. If he started using testosterone, his own production system would wither away. He would become infertile, and he would be dependent on testosterone for the rest of his life. For men whose testosterone has declined because of aging (andropause), hCG would not work to raise testosterone. For them, testosterone replacement therapy would be the best hormone replacement option to bring testosterone levels up.

HCG is used extensively for weight loss and is highly successful in rapid weight loss. Please read our book, "Secrets about the HCG Diet,"[3] to learn more about this weight-loss protocol.

HCG is also used to raise testosterone in men like Ted, whose brains are not producing enough LH to stimulate the testes to produce enough testosterone. To raise LH sufficiently requires ten times the amount of hCG used in the hCG weight loss protocol. The hCG was more expensive and difficult to use than testosterone supplementation. But if Ted wanted to maintain his fertility, this would be the best choice. Careful medical management would be necessary during this time.

Ted chose to do the hCG protocol.

Lowering Ted's estrogen.
To lower Ted's estrogen in a hurry, I started Ted on a prescription of Anastrazole. Anastrazole lowers estrogen by decreasing the enzyme, aromatase. Aromatase turns testosterone into estrogen. We will adjust the dosage as time goes by to keep his estrogen levels in a healthy range.

Ted also decreased his estrogen using these strategies:
1. Lose fat.
   - Eat live foods.
   - Healthy diet.
   - Exercise.
2. Decrease the reabsorption of estrogen in the intestines.
   - Treat dysbiosis with probiotics and avoid antibiotics.
   - Improve intestinal cleansing.
3. Clear xenoestrogens (environmental estrogens) from the body.
   - Detoxify. Read "Secrets to Lose Toxic Belly Fat! Heal Your Sick Metabolism Using State-Of-The-Art Medical Testing and Treatment With Detoxification, Diet, Lifestyle, Supplements, and Bioidentical Hormones." [4]
   - Zeolite.
4. Improve liver function and estrogen clearance.
   - Decrease alcohol.

- Use milk thistle.

- Use Calcium D-Glucarate.

- Do a liver-gall bladder cleanse. For details, read our book, "Keto Smart."[5]

5. Improve estrogen metabolism.

- Use DIM.

Raising Ted's Growth Hormone.

Because testing showed a mild growth hormone insufficiency, we started with the safest methods of raising growth hormone. Ted's improved diet and exercise program was a big help to his growth hormone status. He also started using a non-prescription growth hormone supplement at bedtime (oral secretagogue). He was able to get this supplement in the mail. This was all that Ted needed to bring his growth hormone up into the healthy range. For more detailed information, read our book, "Secrets About Growth Hormone." [6]

Ted's health continued to get better.

His depression improved. This helped in all areas of his life. His marital relationship improved dramatically. Ted began to feel empowered, sexual, and his depression and irritability were relieved, even though stress at work still remained.

Part of Ted's treatment plan is to continue working to heal his adrenals. Because it took many years for his adrenals to become so dysfunctional, it will take time to heal them.

He is to continue on hCG for testosterone replacement as long as it is producing the testosterone elevations that are optimal for him.

The cause for the low LH levels was not evident in our initial testing. But further testing using heavy metal chelation tests found mercury toxicity. Mercury toxicity is a prime suspect in low LH.

I referred Ted to a biological dentist to have the source of the mercury toxicity removed. Ted had a mouth full of silver fillings. These toxic, mercury-containing fillings had been put there by a dentist who was not conscious of or not concerned about the disastrous health consequences of his actions.

For a complete discussion of mercury fillings and other dangerous dental practices, read our book, "TOXIC TEETH: How a Biological (Holistic) Dentist Can Help You Cure Cancer, Facial Pain, Autoimmune, Heart, and Other Disease Caused By Infected Gums, Root Canals, Jawbone Cavitations, and Toxic Metals." [7]

Next, we began a protocol to remove the mercury from Ted's body. If we are able to get the mercury burden down low enough within three years, Ted might be able to raise his testosterone into the normal range without having to use supplemental hormones. By avoiding using testosterone supplementation, he will also avoid the side effects of sterility and shrinking testicles.

Ted began to religiously follow a mercury detoxification program that includes daily use of a far-infrared sauna and supplements. Instructions are detailed in our book, "Secrets to Lose Toxic Belly Fat! Heal Your Sick Metabolism Using State-Of-The-Art Medical Testing and Treatment With Detoxification, Diet, Lifestyle, Supplements, and Bioidentical Hormones."

We will continue to monitor his blood sugar and hormones and make changes to his treatment program as necessary to keep all of his hormones within healthy ranges.

Cheryl gets pregnant and is happy about it.

A year later, Ted's wife, Cheryl, finally got pregnant. They had a healthy baby girl. Ted reports that Cheryl has stopped complaining and that they are much happier.

CHAPTER 3. WHY BOTHER BALANCING HORMONES?

If you want to enjoy optimal emotional and physical health, balancing all of your hormones is essential.

- Hormone imbalances cause many diseases.

- Optimal levels of testosterone are necessary for health.

- Symptoms of low testosterone include poor immunity, loss of muscle mass, decreased bone density, poor mood and memory, getting fatter, losing fitness, loss of potency and libido.

- Low testosterone can kill you in many ways.

- Testosterone levels drop as men get older.

- And testosterone levels are dropping in all men of all ages all over the world. This is probably due to environmental pollution.

Hormone imbalances cause diseases.

- **In the skin,** disease appears as wrinkles, dryness, rashes, and growths.

- **In the brain,** diseases may show up as depression, moodiness, anxiety, forgetfulness, stroke, dementia,[8] or Alzheimer's. Sleep is disturbed.

- **In the joints,** the disease is called arthritis. Lower levels of testosterone often precede rheumatoid arthritis.[9]

- **In the pancreas,** the diseases are called insulin resistance, metabolic syndrome, or type-2 diabetes.[10]

- **In the bones,** the disease is first called osteopenia. As bone disease progresses and bones become even more porous, it is called osteoporosis. Your bones may break. A broken hip can kill you.[11]

- **In the ears,** the disease is called deafness (senile hearing loss).[12]

- **In the eyes,** the disease is called blindness, caused by cataracts or macular degeneration.[13] [14]

- **In the heart and blood vessels,** the diseases are called arrhythmias, atherosclerosis, stroke, or heart failure.[15]

- **In the immune system,** the diseases are cancer and infections.[16]

Treating your hormone imbalances may save your life. A *lack* of vital hormones, like testosterone and growth hormone, as well as an *excess* of other hormones, like estrogen and insulin, leads to the development of diseases that kill men.[17] [18] [19] [20] [21] [22] Hormone imbalances produce a weak immune system, our cancer surveillance system. When hormone balance is disrupted, the risk of prostate and other types of cancer rises.[23] [24] Optimizing your hormones decreases risk of colon cancer,[25] Alzheimer's,[26] dementia,[27] insulin resistance, and diabetes.[28]

Optimal testosterone levels are needed for health:

- Robust erections.
- Plenty of sex drive.
- Building muscles.
- Burning fat.
- Keeping energy up.
- Mood good.
- Immune function strong.
- High bone density.

Symptoms of low testosterone in men:

- **You become grumpy** when you don't have enough testosterone. You get anxious, depressed, and grouchy.
- **You feel tired a lot.**
- **Your competitive drive diminishes.** You lose your motivation, your edge.
- **You have more stiffness and pain in muscles and joints.** Testosterone helps to decrease chronic inflammation.[29]
- **Your fitness drops.** Even if you work out hard in the gym, you just can't build much muscle. Without sufficient testosterone, you can't use the protein that you eat to make muscle.

- **You get fat.**[30] As muscles waste away, fat takes their place. Metabolic rate decreases.[31]
- **Pubic and armpit hair thins out.**
- **Visible changes appear.** As testosterone drops, a man will get wrinkles and get shorter in height, due to the **loss of bone density** and weakened connective tissue. Skin gets dry, thin, and non-elastic, with thin lips, droopy eyelids, and sagging cheeks.
- **The immune system weakens** with decreased ability to detect cancer and fight infectious disease.

Libido and potency decreases: [32]

Sexual problems occur with loss of self-esteem and deteriorating marital relationships. A man's sexual arousal, desire, fantasies and performance go right out the window.

- **Forget the morning erections.** And it takes a lot longer to get it up, when you do. Erections do not occur with fantasies or sight, but require physical stimulation. Erections are not as firm.
- **The need to have orgasm diminishes or disappears.** There is longer recovery time between orgasms. The force of ejaculation is less. The desire for and frequency of masturbation decreases.
- **Performance anxiety is common.** The fear of being able to perform sexually may cause avoidance of sex. Avoidance of sex and loss of self-esteem both result in *further* loss of testosterone.
- **Men may not be able to get hard enough to perform.** Erectile dysfunction is the inability to obtain and maintain an erection sufficient for sexual intercourse.
- **Testes may shrink and sperm count may drop.** The testicles shrink and don't bunch up as much when sexually aroused.

Low testosterone can kill you.[33]

- Low testosterone ages the heart and leads to heart disease.

- Low testosterone ages the brain, decreasing memory and intelligence. Men with low testosterone have more dementia and Alzheimer's.[34]
- Low testosterone also affects the bones, teeth, eyes, and immune system.

Testosterone declines with age in every man.

Now here's the really scary part. The average testosterone levels of American men of all ages are dropping to extremely low levels.[35] The same thing is found in men all over the world. No matter where you check, the average man's testosterone levels are lower than they were in the past.[36] This book gives you strategies to optimize your testosterone levels, no matter how old you are.

Andropause or "manopause" happens when the male sex hormones (androgens) become deficient as a man ages. Some men experience this decline in androgens earlier than others. But all men will be affected sooner or later. Testosterone decline usually begins in the early 30's and drops severely with age.[37] By the age of 80, a man's testosterone level is often only 20% of what it was in his youth.

This hormone drop-off is so sneaky that many men do not even notice it. It is nothing like the sudden drama that many women are thrown into at menopause. But whether he realizes it is happening or not, male sex hormone loss can devastate any man's health.

Why are testosterone levels dropping?

We don't know why, but our best guess is that this is being caused by environmental pollution. Toxins that act like estrogen (a female sex hormone) are at the top of the suspect list of causes for dropping testosterone in men all over the planet.[38] Testosterone may also drop with too much stress,[39] the use of anabolic steroids,[40] depression,[41] smoking,[42] recreational drug use,[43] excessive alcohol use,[44] bad diet,[45] or exposure to harmful chemicals.[46] Many medications elevate the hormone, prolactin, which lowers testosterone.

Medications that raise prolactin include antidepressants, opiates, anticonvulsants, antihypertensives, antihistamines, and antipsychotics.

Next, let's listen to Sam's story of hormonal imbalance. Like Ted, he is a relatively young man who is experiencing symptoms of testosterone deficiency. Also like Ted, his problems were overcome by correcting the cause of the testosterone deficiency.

CHAPTER 4. SAM IS FAT, TIRED, AND DEPRESSED.

Sam is a 45-yr old white male complaining of fatigue, weight gain, loss of muscle mass, poor libido, and decreased sexual performance. Sam says, "My biggest problem is severe depression."

I ask him, "When did all this begin?"

He said, "These problems have been coming on slowly over the past 5-10 years. I was initially diagnosed by my primary-care physician as having a severe depressive disorder. I tried a number of anti-depressants. These all made me feel much worse. I was sent to an internal medicine specialist who diagnosed low thyroid. I was told that my TSH (thyroid stimulating hormone) was quite low. However, when they gave me thyroid hormone, I felt so tired that I couldn't get out of bed."

Sam's history includes a brain injury.

Sam's history is that 15 years ago he was crossing the street in the crosswalk on his bicycle. He was not seen by the driver of the armored car that hit him. He was knocked off of his bicycle. He didn't have any broken bones and had his helmet on, but he was knocked unconscious for a few moments. He states that he has never been right since then. He received the diagnoses of mild traumatic brain injury and has seen excellent therapists, including getting neuro-biofeedback. He has severe problems with multi-tasking (mild traumatic brain injury symptoms).

Labs were normal except for a low TSH.

I reviewed the lab that he presented, which showed normal tests for liver, kidney, CBC, and cholesterol. The primary abnormality was a low TSH. He had no other blood tests or evaluations of his hormones. I recommended that we do laboratory testing for his major hormones and that we evaluate after that. I ordered a four-point cortisol, total and free testosterone, total and free T4, total and free T3, TSH, FSH, LH, and IGF-1.

Sam's cortisol tests show adrenal problems.

The 4-point cortisol testing was returned showing no peak at 8 am and a flat line that drifted down throughout the day. His total and free testosterone levels were in the lower quarter and the total and free T4 and the total and free T3 were in the lower quarter of the reference range. FSH and LH were within normal limits. IGF-1 was in the upper 25th percentile of the reference range.

Diagnosis: Adrenal exhaustion.

Diagnosis: Stage 4 adrenal dysfunction secondary to sluggish pituitary secondary to mild traumatic brain injury.

What this means is that Sam's pituitary gland in his brain had probably been injured in the bike accident. The pituitary could no longer secrete enough ACTH (Adrenocorticotropic Hormone) to stimulate the adrenals to work properly. Thus, his brain was not secreting enough hormone to stimulate his adrenals to secrete enough cortisol hormone to keep him feeling healthy and well.

Cortisol replacement brings fast improvement.

I tell Sam, "If this diagnosis is correct, then replacing your cortisol will bring you great benefit within 24 hours. It is called low-dose cortisol treatment."

I gave him 5 mg of Cortef four times a day. Within 24 hours, his sense of well-being improved tremendously.

Sam's brain has been permanently injured and he will need to be on low-dose cortisol therapy (Cortef) for the rest of his life. His brain will never be able to properly stimulate the adrenals to provide what his body needs. There are no adverse effects from taking low-dose cortisol and the benefits are lifesaving.

I explained to Sam, "To absolutely confirm the diagnosis, we need to do a blood test at 8 am to see if ACTH has its normal 8 am spike. This spike is important for the body's circadian rhythm. The lack of an 8 am spike indicates a brain dysfunction causing adrenal atrophy rather than adrenal burnout. "

The lab results came back showing an 8 am spike in cortisol. So now Sam could begin to heal his adrenals. Just as in Ted's case, I outlined the plan for Sam to heal his adrenals. I explained to Sam that without lifestyle changes, his adrenals could not heal. It is important for him to have a lifelong commitment to adrenal health. Just like Ted, Sam needs to follow the five steps to heal his adrenals.

Let's review the steps to heal the adrenals again, because these steps are important to all of us. In today's stressed-out world, most of us are dealing with less-than-optimal adrenal function.

To heal his adrenals, Sam needed to:

(1) Change his diet.

(2) Get moderate daily exercise.

(3) Take adaptogens (herbs that heal adrenals).

(4) Normalize his sleep.

(5) Slow down his driven attitude and de-stress his life.

NEXT comes thyroid and testicular optimization.

Without enough stress hormones coming from the adrenals, his other hormones could not work well. Just healing the adrenals would allow all of his other hormones to work better.

The reason he felt so horrible when he was given thyroid hormone, even though he was hypothyroid, is that his stress hormones were so depleted that when thyroid hormone increased the metabolism, the body's machinery began to break down. It's like running an engine without oil.

Unfortunately this type of thing happens quite frequently. The conventionally-trained physician, who does not understand how the hormones interact, gives the patient thyroid hormone without even checking adrenal function.

The same thing happened when Sam's physicians prescribed a number of anti-depressants to medicate his depression. None of these medications worked because the underlying cause of Sam's depression was not being addressed.

Sam's condition improves.

Once we corrected the adrenal dysfunction, the function of thyroid hormone and testosterone naturally improved. Once we had the adrenals supported, we then worked to optimize thyroid and testicular function. In Sam's case, his thyroid and testosterone levels normalized.

Now that we have listened to the stores of two young men with testosterone deficiency, let's examine the common problem of low testosterone coming from aging (andropause), then we will listen to John's story of andropause and how we were able to help him, even though his regular doctor refused to treat him for low testosterone.

CHAPTER 5. ARE YOU LOSING YOUR VIRILITY?

No man likes to admit or even suspect that he may be losing his vitality. Andropause may be just as devastating to a man's health and well-being as menopause may be for a woman. But a man is less likely to admit that it is really happening. For this reason, men are much less likely than women to seek treatment for symptoms of low hormone levels.

His partner, however, may be painfully aware of the signs of aging in her mate. He is grumpy. He can't remember things as well. He is falling asleep in his chair after dinner. And sex, if and when it happens at all, just isn't what it used to be. The flame has gone out.

She may be happy with this arrangement if she, too, has deficient sex hormones. If both spouses are hormonally-deficient, then their sex drives will be more matched.

Problems occur when one spouse corrects sex hormone deficiencies and the other does not. If one spouse replaces hormones and the other ignores symptoms of deficient hormones, sex drives may become unmatched.

Consider getting evaluated for hormone imbalances at the same time as your partner. It works best to match sex drives in both partners. Otherwise, one or the other may seek to get their sexual needs met outside the relationship.

It is not unusual for one partner to bring the other along to the doctor's appointment. If a wife brings her husband's health issues up at her doctor visit, her physician may be able to help her husband recognize that andropause has cast a shadow on his health and the health of their relationship. Or a husband may bring his wife along when he goes to see the doctor. Once the situation is acknowledged, an evaluation and treatment program for both partners may work miracles.

Behavior changes as male sex hormones drop.

He becomes more docile and more feminine in nature. Less testosterone and more estrogen also result in the loss of his vital competitive edge and decision-making ability. When a man's testosterone drops, he may try to raise his testosterone temporarily with many different strategies.

Winning is a way to raise testosterone. Testosterone-deficient males may feel like they have lost the battle of life to younger, more powerful males. The testosterone-deficient male looks for any small victory to help bring up his testosterone, perhaps picking fights with his family and co-workers.

Another way that a man may try to raise his testosterone levels is by enhancing his status. A man's car is a symbol of his success in the world. He might buy an expensive SUV, a red convertible sports car, or a Harley to temporarily boost his testosterone levels.

Dying the grey hair away might help him look younger. Scalp implants or a toupee may give the illusion of youth.

An affair with a younger woman would prove that he hasn't lost his virility. Having more sex would certainly raise his testosterone and his self-esteem.

But none of these strategies works in the long run to raise his testosterone. He may become self-destructive, perhaps taking up smoking if he doesn't smoke already, drinking more alcohol, or taking drugs to ease his psychological pain. The worst-case scenario ends in suicide.

Relationship challenges.

Older women may become bossier and older men may let the women boss them around. As a man loses testosterone and estrogen rises, female hormones begin to outweigh male hormones. When this happens, a man typically becomes less aggressive and loses motivation.[47]

The opposite is true for women. As a woman's hormone balance changes at menopause, she may become more domineering and less feminine. As her estrogen drops, a woman's male sex hormones (like testosterone) become greater when compared to her female hormones. This is called androgen dominance.

If a man's wife is menopausal and she is not replacing her lost female sex hormones, the relationship power dynamics may shift. She may become the dominant partner, taking over the decision-making. The combination may work out . . . or it may not.

Sexual problems may occur. If his wife has more androgens than estrogen, she may become demanding, irritable, and disinterested in sex. Vaginal dryness and tissue thinning may make sex painful for the menopausal woman.[48]

Sexual desire and performance decline when a man's male sex hormones decline.[49] Erections may become impossible.[50] Orgasm frequency declines in both men and women.[51]

Both sexes are affected by depression and foul mood. His grumpiness may become unbearable. As she becomes depressed,[52] she may wish to be alone. If the man with low testosterone stays in his relationship, his libido is down, and he feels anxious and alone.

If he doesn't regularly touch his wife, her levels of the hormone, oxytocin, drop. When her levels of oxytocin drop, she may feel lonely and abandoned. Her feelings cause even more anxiety and feelings of isolation in him.

Their relationship may be in trouble. They may struggle on like this for years. But things never seem to be quite as good as they used to be. Relationships become difficult when either one or both of the partners are missing the hormones needed to stabilize moods, ensure health, and allow for great sex.[53]

It is important for both spouses to notice hormone changes in themselves and in each other. In order to feel at their best, they must both be willing to seek out advice from a knowledgeable doctor who is committed to treating mild and moderate hormone imbalances before they become severe.

Three types of low testosterone.

Optimal range for testosterone replacement varies between primary-care physicians and anti-aging doctors. Conservative physicians would target a testosterone level appropriate for age. Anti-aging doctors usually view the levels of a healthy 30-year old man as optimal for every age man and aim for blood levels of testosterone to be in the 800's rather than the 400's.

Hypogonadal.

Men who have been diagnosed as being "hypogonadal" *have testosterone levels that are very low (less than 300 ng/dl).* Most doctors will treat men who have been diagnosed as hypogonadal.

Subclinical.

Patients with a "subclinical" drop in testosterone have testosterone levels above 300 ng/dl, but less than the optimal levels in the 800's. They have underlying pathology, and over time they will eventually decline to hypogonadal levels (less than 300). It is superior medicine to find these patients and treat them when they have mild or moderate hormonal failure and not wait until they have severe disease and reach the hypogonadal level.

Suboptimal.

In patients who have "suboptimal" levels of testosterone, their testosterone level is lower than is optimal for them. Like the subclinical men, their testosterone is above 300 ng/dl.

They differ from the "subclinical" patients, because they do not have pathology that will make their testosterone drop even more. Over time, their testosterone may remain low, but they will not deteriorate to hypogonadal levels, like the subclinical men will. If the man with suboptimal levels of hormones makes lifestyle changes and improves his health, he can raise his testosterone levels back to a healthy level.

Most doctors will not treat either subclinical or suboptimal testosterone deficiencies. Anti-aging doctors will treat all types of testosterone deficiencies.

What is man-o-pause (andropause)?

THE NAME OF THE PAUSE THAT ALL MEN GO THROUGH AS THEY AGE IS CALLED ANDROPAUSE. You may hear it called male menopause or man-o-pause.   Andropause is the medical term for the transition that men go through when androgens (male sex hormones) fall off (pause) as they age.

The word, andropause, didn't even come into existence until 1944.[54] Before that, the average man died before getting old enough to experience a significant drop in male hormones. Until the twentieth century, people died younger, because they didn't have any of the modern medical miracles that we now take for granted.

In this day and age, most men do live long enough to experience andropause. But as a man's lifespan increases and testosterone levels drop, his health worsens and disease increases.

Treating andropause is treating a deficiency disease. Androgens (like testosterone and DHEA) and growth hormone (GH) are important hormones that may become deficient as a man ages.

Some men may be able to bring their testosterone levels up just by improving their lifestyle habits[55] and using supplements. Other men may find that the keys to outrageously fantastic health are to use prescription hormones.

But getting a prescription may be tricky. Read on to get advice on how to find a doctor who will write that prescription for you when it is needed to treat testosterone deficiency.

CHAPTER 6. JOHN WANTS A SECOND OPINION.

Next, let's listen to John's andropausal story. John wants a second opinion, because the conventional medical system is not helping him.

JOHN IS A 63-YEAR OLD MAN WHO WOULD LIKE A SECOND OPINION ABOUT HIS TESTOSTERONE. He saw his family doctor six months ago for complaints about feeling weak, tired, and loss of interest in life.

Conventional medical doctors haven't helped.

John told me, "My family doctor sent me to an endocrinologist, a specialist in testosterone, and he did blood tests. The endocrinologist told me that my total testosterone was fine for my age, at 350. He said my free testosterone was in the low normal range. He also noted that my cholesterol was elevated from five years ago and the white blood cell count is low normal. The specialist said I was just getting older. He said he would see me in a year and re-check the testosterone."

The endocrinologist told him, "In the meantime, exercise and eat well."

John exclaimed, "I ALREADY do that!"

John's history indicates hormone problems.

John explained to me that, "The endocrinologist's inability to help me sent me looking for another doctor who might be able to give me some useful advice. A friend of mine told me about how you, Dr. Swartz, helped him to begin to feel better. I decided to get your opinion."

I begin with John's history.

John denies feeling depressed. He does have stress in his relationship with his wife. He lost his interest in sex a few years ago, and his wife isn't interested either. He misses the intimacy, but doesn't think about sex anymore.

His wife has changed since she became menopausal. She has gained weight, has gotten very bossy, and has dark hair on her upper lip. She has no interest in sex.

John has worked out daily for years and especially likes weight lifting. But he complains that he tires so much faster now and has had to lower his weights compared to a year ago. He could always do 20 push-ups, but now barely 12.

John complains that, "I always work out hard, but I just can't gain strength. My joints injure more easily, as well. I get colds easier, and they last longer. The cough just won't go away like it used to."

Screening for hormones and bone density is needed.

After my exam, I told John, "We need to check for the complications of low testosterone to know whether 350 is adequate for YOU or if it is a hormonal deficiency." I explain to John that, "The first blood test we need to determine if this is true testosterone deficiency or not is to check the brain's stimulation of the testes by measuring luteinizing hormone (LH).

If LH is highly elevated, this would indicate that you have failure of the cells in the testes producing testosterone. It is the most common cause of testosterone deficiency in older men."

"We need to order bone density testing, as well. I am most concerned about osteoporosis. Osteoporosis, a preventable, but untreatable disease can often result from low testosterone. Low testosterone not only causes loss of muscle mass, but weak bones.You may be more vulnerable to illnesses because the immune system is weaker in low testosterone states, and there is increased hardening of the arteries.

"Frailty syndrome occurs when an elderly person loses muscle mass, bone mass, proper functioning of the immune system, and neurologic problems. If the bone scan should show osteoporosis, then we need to evaluate for the other possible causes of frailty syndrome, like adult growth hormone deficiency. We also need to do a screening blood test for thyroid function and adrenal function."

Tests show low bone density, high LH, and adrenal dysfunction.

The bone density scan shows severe osteopenia, being very close to osteoporosis. The blood test for growth hormone (IGF-1) is normal.

Four-point adrenal testing shows stage 3 dysfunction, indicating early adrenal burn-out. The testing for adrenal hormone in the morning, noon, afternoon, and midnight shows a drop during the day, indicating prolonged stress on the adrenals. Thyroid tests (total and free T-4, a total and free T-3, and the TSH) were within normal limits.

LH is highly elevated. I told John, "Your diagnosis is that you have primary testicular failure, progressing from moderately severe to severe hypogonadism (testosterone deficiency)."

"FROM AN ANTI-AGING PERSPECTIVE, THE HIGH ELEVATION OF LH TELLS US FOR CERTAIN THAT YOUR BODY'S LEVEL OF TESTOSTERONE OF 350 IS INADEQUATE AND IS A STATE OF DEFICIENCY." This is subclinical low testosterone.

"In a state of subclinical hormonal deficiency, your body weakens with time, allowing the body to age much faster. You are more prone to infections, have hardening of the arteries that is proceeding at a more rapid rate, as well as brain dysfunction from the effect of low testosterone on the brain."

The longer you persist in this state, the worse things will become, so the anti-aging doctor is eager to treat mild and moderate hormonal dysfunction before it becomes severe. Anti-aging doctors differ in their opinions on the appropriate treatment for testosterone before it drops below the lowest reference value (300). Traditionally-trained endocrinologists believe that you only treat the low testosterone after it drops below this reference value. The specialist is practicing standard-of-care for this problem in his specialty.

Anti-aging doctors are trained to diagnose and treat mild and moderate hormonal dysfunction BEFORE it becomes severe. Your testosterone will most assuredly drift down to the magic 300 number over the next one year or five years, if things continue as they are.

"The only treatment option is supplemental testosterone, either by injection, pellets, or topical. There are dangers from testosterone replacement therapy, but the dangers are much greater to not have supplemental testosterone therapy when you are hormonally-deficient.

The dangers of not treating testosterone deficiency are great indeed. Hypogonadal males are at increased risk for death from all causes—accidents, cancer, heart attack, stroke."

THE TREATMENT I RECOMMEND FOR JOHN IS BIOIDENTICAL TESTOSTERONE, EITHER TOPICAL OR BY INJECTION.

We need to get a baseline hemoglobin hematocrit and check that every six months for a year. We will also need a baseline PSA, as well as a fasting blood sugar. We will have to initially evaluate testosterone levels and adjust the dosage appropriately.

The highest priority is treatment of the osteopenia and to prevent progression. There are more blood tests that might be done, but the keys to correcting low bone density are weight-bearing exercise and a diet free of processed food." You can only begin testosterone treatment understanding the risks, benefits, and the necessary medical monitoring.

Risks—shrinking testicles, feminization.

The major concern with testosterone therapy is that within a relatively short period of time you will have testicular atrophy and withering (shrinking balls). You will become progressively infertile.

The complications of testosterone therapy can be polycythemia (elevation of the red blood cell count) which can be very serious. You can get a blood clot and die.

Testosterone is converted into either DHT or estradiol.

- DHT elevations will encourage male pattern baldness and prostate congestion.
- Estrogen elevation causes gynocomastia (bitch tits), weight gain, and feminization of the male.

Benefits—strength, thinking, sex drive.

The benefits of supplemental testosterone are:

- You will rapidly begin gaining muscle and strength.
- Your mind will become brighter.
- Your libido will return. Depression will lift.
- Your immune system will be significantly stronger. You will resist and heal infections much faster.
- Hardening of the arteries will progress at a slower rate.

Adrenal treatment—decrease stress.

To treat the stage 3 adrenal dysfunction, I encouraged John to decrease the stress in his life--physical, mental, and emotional. The testosterone deficiency is such a great stress on every system of the body that correcting the testosterone deficiency will, by itself, correct the adrenal dysfunction.

John responded immediately.

John followed the program and he immediately gained muscle mass and strength, had better libido, and felt brighter in his outlook on life.

John's wife may need hormone treatment.

I explain to John that, "At this point it may be wise for your wife to consider bioidentical hormone replacement to avoid destabilization of your relationship." Now that John has corrected his testosterone deficiency, he may be tempted to seek satisfaction of his sexual needs outside the marital relationship if his menopausal wife is unwilling to participate.

Many men are suffering from symptoms caused by high levels of the female sex hormone, estrogen.　Let's examine that common problem and listen to Ben's story of elevated estrogen and low testosterone.

CHAPTER 7. HIGH ESTROGEN = BEER BELLIES AND MAN BOOBS.

Estrogen is important for a male, just as it is for a female. Not only is it important for maintaining strong bones, it is important to the brain, and for erectile function. Estrogen is essential for the new growth of neurons, as well as the maintenance of healthy neurons.

But too much estrogen is a big problem for men. 80% of a man's estrogen is made in his abdominal fat cells. 20% of the estrogen comes from the testes. We know that benign prostatic hyperplasia (BPH) incidence increases with age. DHT, estradiol, and estrone accumulate in the prostate with aging. Research is showing that a reason for this is testosterone dropping as estrogen increases.[56]

As male sex hormone and growth hormone levels drop, levels of the female sex hormone, estrogen, go up. Too much estrogen in men has become a big problem, contributing to weight problems and obesity.

Andropausal men have much more estrogen in relation to their testosterone than they did when they were younger. These estrogen-dominant andropausal men become feminized, less aggressive, and are more easily bossed around by their menopausal wives.

More men of all ages are getting "beer bellies" and "man boobs." As estrogen rises in a man, his belly gets fatter and begins to overflow his belt. There is no hope of ever getting a six-pack. No amount of sit-ups and crunches can fix this problem. You have to fix the sick metabolism and balance the hormones.

As estrogen rises and testosterone drops, men become more feminine. Enzymes (aromatases) in belly fat take testosterone and turn it into estrogen. Men need some estrogen. But too much estrogen is not good. These men often develop a "beer belly." The added estrogen makes them fat and also causes female-like breasts. As estrogen rises, a man's chest loses its virile look and begins to resemble the female chest. This is happening to more and more men, both young and old. "Gynecomastia" means increased breast tissue in a man. Compare the shapes of men that you see today with those that you see in films or pictures that were recorded years ago. Men used to be slimmer and sexier. The average man today has more estrogen and less testosterone than the average man of past generations.

The beer belly and man boobs are danger signs that a man's health is declining. This rise in estrogen may lead to metabolic syndrome (pre-diabetes), type 2 diabetes, and prostate problems (benign prostatic hypertrophy--BPH and prostate cancer).[57]

High estrogen, poor estrogen metabolism lead to strokes & cancer.

When estrogen levels get too high in relation to testosterone, a man is said to be "estrogen-dominant." In women, estrogen dominance means too much estrogen in relation to progesterone, but in men, estrogen dominance is too much estrogen in relation to testosterone.

When we can't properly metabolize hormones, especially estrogen, we become more susceptible to diseases, especially cancer.[58] Estrogen, like all hormones and drugs, is metabolized primarily in the liver to be safely removed from the body. If your body breaks down estrogen into the ugly metabolite, 16-OH estrone, your risk for prostate and other cancers increases.

The estrogen-dominant environment is cancer-friendly in both men and women. Estrogen builds things up. This excessive tissue growth happens in the estrogen-dominant female and in the estrogen-dominant male. In men, too much estrogen in relation to testosterone can cause cancer, including prostate cancer.[59][60][61]

Excess estrogen promotes abnormal blood clotting.[62] The most common cause of stroke is clotting in the blood vessels of the brain. Men with the highest blood levels of estrogen have over twice the risk for stroke.[63]

Where does the excess estrogen come from?

As levels of environmental pollution increase, so do estrogen levels in everybody. The problem is especially bad in water from wastewater treatment plants (tap water). The fish in these waters are so loaded up with estrogen that there are more females than males.[64]

Estrogen levels in both men and women are the result of the sum of the estrogen our bodies make, the estrogens in our diet and water, the estrogen metabolites (produced when estrogen is broken down), and the estrogen-like chemicals (the xenoestrogens) that we have absorbed into our bodies from the environment. Wastewater treatment plants dump huge amounts of estrogen into the water. The estrogen in the wastewater comes from the waste products of women on birth control pills, as well as both women AND gay men who take supplemental estrogen. The massive amounts of pesticides, herbicides, shampoos, detergents, soaps, prescription and non-prescription drugs, and other chemicals dumped into the water act like estrogen and are called xenoestrogens. Drinking and bathing in tap water just adds to the xenoestrogen burden of men, women, and children.

We all ingest large amounts of xenoestrogens from the water, food, and environment. These xenoestrogens contribute greatly to the problem of estrogen dominance. Toxic chemicals are absorbed right through the skin. These estrogen-mimickers raise the body's estrogen load, increasing cancer risk. Many skin products may disrupt hormone balance. They often contain DHEA and pregnenolone, which can raise estrogen levels. Those who play golf breathe in the chemicals used on the golf course. We all drink chemicals in our groundwater. Plastics are another major source of xenoestrogens. If you eat meat, unless you make it a point to eat organic meat, you will ingest synthetic hormones that were fed to the animals to increase their growth rate. The herbicides and insecticides used on the plant world are concentrated in the animal fat. We concentrate these toxins further when we ingest them.

A major concern is that these xenoestrogens are excreted from the body only in very small amounts. They not only accumulate over a lifetime, but avidly bind to the cells' estrogen receptors, usually more avidly than estrogen. Some of them may even bind permanently to the estrogen receptors and forever block the cells' ability to take in bioidentical estrogen.

Keep trim and correct faulty estrogen metabolism.

To stay healthy a man needs to keep trim. That beer belly is not healthy for a man. You want to reduce the belly fat because it produces an enzyme that turns your testosterone into estrogen. If the enzyme, aromatase (estrogen synthase) is present, testosterone will turn into estrogen. That enzyme is produced by belly fat. Estrogen metabolism can change after andropause. It is wise to get an estrogen metabolism test and then correct faulty estrogen metabolism. Use DIM and detoxify. Follow the advice in "Secrets to Lose Toxic Belly Fat! Heal Your Sick Metabolism Using State-Of-The-Art Medical Testing and Treatment With Detoxification, Diet, Lifestyle, Supplements, and Bioidentical Hormones."[65]

CHAPTER 8. BEN HAS HIGH ESTROGEN.

BEN IS A 45-YEAR OLD BLACK MALE COMPLAINING OF FATIGUE AND IMPAIRED PERFORMANCE, DESPITE INCREASED EFFORT. Ben has been a serious body-builder for 30 years and knows his body very well. He can find no explanation for his decreased weight performance. His diet, he feels, is good with limited processed foods. He takes large amounts of supplements for maximal bodybuilding, and eats lots of vegetables and meats or fish.

Ben had the insidious (coming out of nowhere) onset for the past year of decreased performance in his bodybuilding program. He denies the use of anabolic steroids, but has intermittently used growth hormone products in the past, however, not in the past year.

He consulted a sports doctor who ordered testosterone testing. Ben reports that his total testosterone, as well as his free testosterone were in the lower third of normal (suboptimal).

Sexual history revealed that he has had a lapse of performance over the past year in this area, as well. He rated his sex life as "super" until the past year. He doesn't have the vitality in his erections that he used to.

He is also more inclined to be sedentary and less active. The sports doctor said that he is just getting older.

He is not as motivated for sexual activity as he has been in the past and therefore he doesn't initiate sexual activity as often.

Ben tells me, "My wife wanted me to come, because she would like 'me' back. I think my wife is too dominating, and that is the problem."

Fertility is an issue. He is therefore not a candidate for testosterone replacement.

Why is Ben's testosterone level low? The question is, "Why are his gonads failing?" The pituitary is appropriately trying to stimulate the production of testosterone, but it can't happen. Getting older is no explanation for pathology. If he waits long enough, he will continue to drop his testosterone toward a true hypogonadal level, and his health will deteriorate during that time, compared to having optimal hormone present.

Initial lab tests point to elevated estrogen.

I ordered a lab: an LH, estradiol, DHT, IGF-1, total and free testosterone, SHBG, hematocrit, and PSA. The lab values show a marked elevation in estrogen, DHT within normal limits, LH is mildly elevated, and normal Growth Hormone.

The diagnosis is elevated estrogen with early primary hypogonadism, benign prostatic hypertrophy secondary to elevated estrogen.

Lowering Ben's estrogen is the first goal.

The first goal is to correct the elevated estrogen as much as we can, support testosterone production, and remove any xenoestrogens that are causing abnormal estrogen metabolism. It is important that we do estrogen metabolism testing, but testing for toxins that impair testicular production of testosterone is much more difficult. Certainly, phthalates from all plastics and pesticides are potent xenoestrogens, causing abnormal and prolonged stimulation of the estrogen receptor.

Diagnosis: The decreased performance in weight lifting and the fatigue are a result of the elevated estrogen and early declining testosterone.

More tests are needed.

Ben needs estrogen metabolism testing, bone density testing, and evaluation of insulin status. If the bones are shown to be osteopenic, meaning they are beginning to de-mineralize, the mild hypogonadism would be treated much more aggressively.

Ben is not metabolizing estrogen well.

The estrogen metabolism testing shows elevations in the estrogen metabolites that cause cancer, and the good estrogen metabolites to be very low.

Ben is resistant to insulin.

Insulin tests show mild insulin resistance.

"Insulin resistance is a driving force, both for the elevated estrogen and the declining testosterone. Testosterone must become either estrogen or DHT. If we decrease the amount of testosterone being converted to estrogen, we will achieve increased total testosterone levels. In many ways, especially in the mind and genitals, estrogen opposes testosterone. Decreasing estrogen will therefore improve the hormonal performance for testosterone by removing the opposing force.

Eliminating insulin resistance is the key to improvement of your health. Not only will this help hormones normalize, your general health and sense of well-being will significantly improve. Degenerative diseases are reversed as insulin sensitivity returns. Insulin is a highly-inflammatory hormone that can drive inflammation throughout the body when it is elevated.

I told Ben to follow the KetoSmart 10-step program to reverse insulin resistance." [66] On questioning, Ben had the symptoms of normal thyroid function and adrenal function. He states that he is a low-stress guy in a low-stress job. He has had more urination during the night. He used to not go at all in the night, but now has to go one or two times every night. His stream is a little weaker with dribbling at the end.

Ben has low bone density.

Bone density testing comes back mildly osteopenic for age. This is unusual for a weight-lifter. The weak bones are a strong indication for more aggressive treatment.

Detoxifying xenoestrogens is paramount.

I tell Ben, "A general program of detoxification for xenoestrogens would be more important for you than for other people. Please read Secrets to Lose Toxic Belly Fat for detailed information.[67] The overall current plan is to normalize estrogen production by controlling high estrogen with aromatase inhibitors (Anastrozole) and to use DIM to heal abnormal estrogen metabolism. He is to follow the Keto Smart program to heal insulin resistance and aggressively work to detoxify xenoestrogens."

Re-evaluation in three months.

"I would re-evaluate your fatigue and performance after three months of our treatment program. If the performance is improved, as expected, energy returns. Then we know the primary problem has been corrected and continued cleansing of toxins is the most important long-term goal.

Since fertility is important, I would avoid testosterone therapy as long as clinically possible. If testosterone continues to decline after we get the estrogen down, this would produce low sperm production and impaired fertility.

At that point, treatment with clomiphene would give us a few more years of improved sperm production and testicular production of testosterone. Long-term cleansing of chemicals toxic to testicular cells would continue to be important for general health and cancer prevention."

Next, let's consider growth hormone, see what a deficiency looks like, and listen to Fred's story of true growth hormone deficiency.

CHAPTER 9. WHAT ABOUT GROWTH HORMONE?

Growth hormone is also critical for good health and may be low, even in young men. Growth hormone (GH) begins to drop at age thirty. When growth hormone levels drop, the body begins to wither and waste away.[68] The immune system weakens, and you get sick easier. As the bones weaken, they may break. Your muscles get smaller, and you get fatter. Your organs (kidneys, stomach, small intestine, liver, and spleen) shrink.

Growth-hormone deficient men are generally osteopenic or osteoporotic.[69] But true growth hormone deficiency is a rare disorder.

Testosterone and growth hormone work together synergistically to increase strength far more than either one alone could do. Supplementing with testosterone will raise growth hormone secretion.[70]

But if growth hormone levels are really low, testosterone alone is not going to bring growth hormone up enough to make a real difference. So growth hormone deficiency needs to be treated when it is present.

Check GH levels along with all of the other hormones that decline as we age. It's easy to overlook low GH.

If you are deficient in growth hormone, taking growth hormone supplements and/or injectable growth hormone may help you to live longer.[71] Most people at age 60 have growth hormone levels that would be considered to be seriously deficient in a younger person. Produced in the pituitary gland in the brain, growth hormone slows aging, especially cardiovascular disease. Growth hormone does not make adults grow, unless it is present in pathologically high levels, which results in acromegaly.

Growth hormone in the adult could more accurately be called "repair hormone." Growth hormone repairs your brain and your body. Growth hormone works to keep your immune system healthy and your bones and muscles strong. Growth hormone decreases inflammation. Growth hormone keeps you in a good mood, normalizes weight by increasing muscle mass and fat loss, gives you more energy, and helps you to think clearly.

Growth Hormone (GH) decreases beginning at age thirty. As we age, most of us in the U.S. have levels of GH that are too low for optimal health. Aboriginal cultures that live as hunter-gatherers in an environment without toxic pollution don't have these problems. Drop in GH causes decreased bone mass and density, decreased muscle mass, and increased fat by up to 40%. It also causes shrinkage in kidneys, stomach, small intestine, liver, and spleen with decreased immune resilience.

Symptoms of Adult GH Deficiency (AGHD):

- Decreased quantity and quality of life.
- Reduced immunity and healing.
- Chronic fatigue, loss of exercise capacity, loss of endurance.
- Decreased confidence and optimism, lack of drive and vigor.
- Loss of bone strength, osteopenia, osteoporosis (loss of bone density).
- Decreased muscle tone and sarcopenia (loss of muscle mass).
- Increased total and intra-abdominal fat.
- Loss of concentration.
- Anxiety, depressed mood.
- Sexual function disorders.
- Poor sleep.[72]
- Glucose intolerance.
- Increased skin wrinkling and decreased skin thickness, increased fragility of skin and blood vessels.
- Atherosclerosis, increased total cholesterol, LDL cholesterol, and apolipoprotein B.

If a GH decrease is subclinical, your GH is low for you but within normal laboratory limits, and there is pathology present. You will eventually end up in AGHD. Subclinical GH decrease produces a mild to moderate frailty syndrome. Anti-aging physicians believe that subclinical low levels of GH should be treated. One or five or ten years from now, it will become true GH deficiency (AGHD), as your GH is headed down, down, down. By the time you have become growth-hormone deficient, your health will have deteriorated significantly.

If GH is suboptimal, it is within normal lab limits, but there isn't the progressive pathology that will lead to AGHD. If GH is drifting down from age, poor health, but not a pathological depression—it is called GH insufficiency. These suboptimal levels of GH mean that GH is low for you for optimal health.   GH level decline may be age-appropriate, meaning you have declining hormone levels as you get older and wear out. But if you had higher, optimal levels, you would be more vital, live longer, age less quickly, build stronger bones and more muscle, and lose fat. Anti-aging physicians treat all suboptimal hormone levels, because optimal hormones equal optimal health and longevity.

Adult Growth Hormone Deficiency (AGHD) is a rare disorder that most physicians will treat, because this is a serious problem. AGHD is identified by IGF-1 levels or urinary GH levels that are below laboratory reference levels. By the strictest definition, any person with IGF-1 levels less than 100 mcg/ml is GH-deficient (AGHD). But many anti-aging experts use anything less than 350 mcg/ml as GH-deficient.

Standard of care for traditional doctors is to wait until IGF-1 values are below the lowest lab values, i.e., extremely GH-deficient, before offering treatment.   By then, you would have deteriorated over however long it took you to drop to the lowest lab values. Atherosclerotic vascular disease, poor immune function, increasing fat, with weakening muscles and bones would be advancing over this period of time.

Anti-aging physicians prefer to treat GH problems before they get to the severe state of AGHD, or when GH decrease is still in the subclinical stage of mild to moderate dysfunction. This is preferable to waiting for five or ten years until the problem becomes severe.

If GH levels are subclinically depressed, treatment can be of great benefit to your health and well-being. Your health would significantly improve if GH were optimized. Many anti-aging professionals recommend that for optimal health, it is wise to bring GH levels back up to those of a healthy 32-year-old. When you get a prescription to treat subclinical growth hormone deficiencies, your doctor is writing an off-label prescription, which means that this medicine is being used to treat a condition that has not been officially approved. Growth hormone is the only drug that has ever been legislated to be illegal for off-label use. So, many doctors are afraid to use growth hormone off label, even though medically, it might be necessary to treat your declining health.[73]

Growth hormone does not cause cancers.[74] **Because it may stimulate the growth of existing cancers, the benefit must greatly outweigh the risk.** In men, studies suggest that the higher the IGF-1 levels, the greater the risk for prostate cancer.[75]

CHAPTER 10. FRED IS GROWTH HORMONE DEFICIENT.

Fred is a 68-year old white male. He complains of weight loss, weakness, and depression. He describes an insidious onset that started a long time ago. He just feels worse and worse.

His doctor diagnosed that he was getting older. Fred states, "I feel like I am an old man and getting senile. I can't do anything anymore. I either wear out or get confused. I don't know if it's my brain or my body."

I ask him about sex. He says, "What's that? It's been so long since I have been interested. My wife kind of lost interest. I was having some erectile problems. It was embarrassing. I tried Viagra, and that helped some, but I still didn't feel that interested. I know I am getting older. My doctor said I have osteoporosis and wants to put me on this drug. I really don't want it, but he says my bones will break if I don't do it."

I ask him, "Did your doctor do any blood tests?"

He says, "Oh yes. He checked it all--my kidneys, my liver, my blood count, my cholesterol. He said I was totally fine, all except for the cholesterol. Then he gave me a statin drug for that."

"Have you had your hormones checked?"

"I am not sure. My doctor didn't say anything, but he was terribly busy. The nurse talked to me about my cholesterol, and then they said that they needed to check a PSA for my prostate. It was normal."

Review of systems:

"We are going to review your hormonal systems and see if there is anything there."

Thyroid screen: Weight lost rather than weight gained appears not to be hypothyroidism. There are no heart palpitations or other symptoms of hyperthyroidism.

Screening questions on the adrenals reveal extremely poor and restless sleep, severe chronic fatigue. He feels wired but tired. Any physical or emotional stress will put him in bed. He has had a high-stress lifestyle and the stress of illness over the past five years has made life much more stressful. He has minimal interest in sex and significant erectile dysfunction.

Reviewing growth hormone, he admits to unintentional weight loss of more than 10 pounds despite adequate nutrition and no reason for a catabolic state. He admits to poor endurance, muscular weakness, low physical activity, and even walking has become slow.

Labs reveal extremely low Growth Hormone.

Lab: His thyroid tests appear normal. Adrenal stage 3 burn-out. IGF-1 is extremely low. LH is low normal. FSH low normal. SHBG is high normal. Total testosterone 360. Free testosterone low normal.

Diagnosis: Adult Growth Hormone Deficiency.

"Your diagnosis is Adult Growth Hormone Deficiency Syndrome. Growth Hormone in adults should be called repair hormone because it maintains healthy tissues. With Adult Growth Hormone Deficiency we need to exclude known possible causes. I would recommend studies to rule out a small tumor in the pituitary (a microadenoma)."

Treatment: gradual growth hormone replacement.

I explain to Fred, "Growth hormone replacement will return you to health. We need to start slowly. It has been many years that you have been deficient. We need to start out at a low dose and slowly increase. We still need to find out why growth hormone is so deficient."

Once growth hormone has been replaced, then we will optimize testosterone, thyroid, and adrenal hormones. We started Fred on Growth hormone replacement.

He is not yet an Olympic champion in weight lifting, but he has been able to begin a resistance training program and is gaining muscles and weight. His depression has lifted, sex drive is coming back, and bone density is increasing.

CHAPTER 11. IMPROVE YOUR LIFESTYLE.

NOW, LET'S LOOK AT LIFESTYLE IMPROVEMENTS YOU CAN MAKE TO GET YOUR HORMONES BACK INTO BALANCE.

Hormones worsen with poor lifestyle.

Jumping immediately into testosterone replacement therapy may not be the best option for treating low testosterone levels. Before you consider how to treat your hormone issues, you need to figure out why you have these issues.

Realize that you are not alone. Many men, even very young men have low testosterone levels. Why are so many of us experiencing hormonal imbalances that were not known to past generations?

Many reasons for hormone imbalances are related to the choices you make about your lifestyle. It works the other way around, too. Your hormones affect your lifestyle. If your hormones are a problem, you are less inclined to choose a healthy lifestyle. You may not choose to exercise, de-stress, and take the time to create healthy meals.

We now face five challenges to our hormones that were unknown to our ancestors:

1) We live in a polluted environment, and many people make their bodies even more polluted by choosing to use drugs, including tobacco and alcohol.

2) We do not receive adequate nutrition (nutrient-depleted soils and our fast-food diets).

3) We are stressed 24-7.

4) We do not get proper exercise.

5) We are living longer.

1) A major cause of hormone imbalance is pollution. Do you live in a natural, unpolluted environment and do not use toxic products on your skin and in your body? Few people can answer yes to that question. Most of us are exposed to massive amounts of environmental toxins that affect our hormones.

Our environment is filled with herbicides, pesticides, heavy metals, radiation, plastics, and chemicals. We are exposed to huge amounts of toxic substances being sprayed and belched into the air from the widespread use of herbicides, pesticides, and jet and auto exhaust, just to name a few of the culprits.

Many people blindly use toxic products on their hair and skin, drink public water, and/or eat the standard American diet (S.A.D.). Vaccinations, root canals, and amalgam (mercury-filled) dental fillings are other major sources of internal pollution.

The use of both legal and illegal drugs, including alcohol, tobacco, and caffeine is another serious way to take in toxins. Prescription and non-prescription drug use is at an all-time high. We even give our children toxic drugs to treat their depression, A.D.D., and other disorders. Children in past times did not need anti-depressants and mood stabilizers.

These toxins make us sick. Any chemicals that contact our skin are absorbed right into our bodies. We also ingest them through our mouths in the food we eat and the water we drink. We breathe them in, too. Then, the blood carries the damaging chemicals to every cell in our bodies.

Toxins block hormones from doing their job. These toxins block our cells from being able to receive the hormones that we need to stay healthy. The hormones knock on the cell doors. But toxins guard the cell doors, like big nasty bouncers refusing to let the hormones come in. The cells then get sick because they are missing vital hormones. A man may be producing plenty of testosterone, but if toxins are blocking the way into the cells, that testosterone can't get into the cells where it is needed to maintain health.

Levels of toxic substances that mimic estrogen (xenoestrogens) are rising in everybody. Our bodies have a very difficult time breaking down and removing these estrogen-mimicking chemicals. Xenoestrogens that come from the toxins in our environment, especially plastics, contribute to a common hormone imbalance that affects men, women, and children.   Much of our food and drink comes in plastic containers.   The different plastics leach into our food and drink.   Many of these poisons attach to estrogen receptors on the cells in our bodies.   These xenoestrogens either block the effect of natural estrogen or create a sick version of receptor stimulation.

All of the toxins that we absorb into our bodies have one thing in common. **They go in, but they never come out.** These thousands of poisons in our modern bodies are carefully stored in the matrix system.   The matrix is the space outside your cells and the space between the capillary bed and the cell.   The poisons are stored in the matrix to keep them away from vital organs, like kidneys and brain, which would be poisoned by them.

As time goes by, the matrix system gets so overloaded with toxins that it can't store any more. When this happens, the toxins may seriously damage vital organs. This is why it is so important to clean the toxins out of the body.

2) Poor nutrition is another big reason for changing hormone levels.[76] Bad diets certainly contribute to the obesity epidemic.[77]   Obesity is a major factor in hormonal imbalances.[78]

Just look at the huge number of fast-food establishments.   Fast food is a relatively new concept that was not in the vocabulary of past generations. Now, there seem to be two or three fast food places on every major corner. Fast food is filled with preservatives, salt, sugar, corn syrup, artificial hormones, trans-fat, saturated fat, and addictive chemicals, like MSG.   It is foodless food.   Regular restaurants are not much better, and you never quite know what you are eating.

Soda pop and ice cream are recent health-destroying substances that were not available to our ancestors. Soda pop creates obesity and cola sodas eat away the bones. The effects of the chemicals in these food substitutes are devastating to our health.   Even so, their use is rampant.

Shelves in the grocery store are filled with processed foods that lack nutrition and overload the body with sodium, sugar, preservatives, and chemicals. Grocery stores may contain a few items of organic produce, but often it was harvested weeks ago and has lost much of its nutritive value. Convenience stores usually don't offer a single item of chemical-free nourishment.

Past generations generally ate much healthier foods. It used to be common for people to grow huge gardens, raise their own chickens, and trade with neighbors for other healthy foods.

Farmers rotated their crops and used natural fertilizers. The soil in which the produce grew was loaded with vitamins and minerals. Cattle only ate grass. Chickens roamed freely. Fish were not poisoned with mercury or raised in toxic conditions on fish farms. At that time, the word "organic" was not in the vocabulary. Everything was organic before herbicides, pesticides, fungicides, antibiotics, and other chemicals permeated the food supply.

Now our bodies must constantly struggle to detoxify the endless toxins in our food supply that cannot be avoided. Some of the chemicals we are eating were originally developed to be used as biological weapons in war. The chemical manufacturers found these biological weapons to be effective in killing insects and plants.

Because ordinary plants will die when sprayed with the herbicides, the chemical manufacturers have now produced genetically-modified plants (GMO) which can withstand being sprayed with massive quantities of these chemical poisons. High levels of these chemical toxins are absorbed into our bodies when we eat foods made from these GMO-modified plants.

To stop the intake of poisonous chemicals in your food, base your diet on organic vegetables and fruits with whole grains, beans, nuts, and seeds. If you eat meat, eat only organic, grass-fed and grass-finished meat. "Natural" does not mean organic. Look for the word, "organic" on the package. Non-organic meat is a concentrated source of toxins.

Health food stores are your best bet for finding nutrition, as they offer the best selection of organic foods that have not been processed. This is the best way to get the nutrients that your body needs to be healthy. To supercharge your health, drink as much fresh vegetable and fruit juice as you can. Fresh (not bottled or canned) juice from organic vegetables and fruits will give your body the nutrients that it needs in an easy-to-assimilate form.

Avoid vegetable oils, such as bottled salad dressings, restaurant salad dressings, and seed oils, such as safflower oil, peanut oil, and corn oil. Many prepared foods have large amounts of these oils. This includes most breads, doughnuts, cookies, crackers, and chips. Other oils to avoid include canola oil, soybean oil, and wheat germ oil. These oils are too high in omega-6 fats.

Avoid bad fats if you want to avoid inflammation and immune system harm. When choosing fats, remember that when omega-6 fats are the predominant fats in your diet, your body will produce hormones that cause inflammation. The standard American diet (S.A.D.) is grossly flooded with these omega-6 fats, found in fast foods and vegetable oils.

To reduce inflammation, consume more omega-3 fats. Olive oil has been proven to be beneficial by the success of the Mediterranean diet. Omega-3 fats are abundant in seafood, such as wild salmon, herring, sardines, mussels, clams, and shrimp.

3) We have too much stress. As a rule, our ancestors lived a quieter, less-stressed life. Most of the things and situations that cause our stress did not exist a hundred years ago.

As we age, it becomes harder to adapt to stress. Each stress takes its toll. All of your little stresses add up. When our nervous systems are under constant stress, it becomes difficult to get enough deep, undisturbed sleep. Without enough quality sleep, we cannot make enough hormones to stay healthy.

If we want to prevent the health decline that results from stress, we can arrange our lives to minimize stress. We can reframe our reactions to stress and maintain a positive outlook. Have an attitude of gratitude. We can let go of our attachment to things that we do not absolutely need and situations that cause us stress. Seek to creatively reduce the negative aspects of your job and relationships. If you have to commute, for example, listen to audiobooks, especially ones that help to improve your life. We cannot balance our hormones with unhealthy stress levels.

4) Fitness is falling. Today we must make an effort to keep fit. Our ancestors didn't need to go to gyms to get their exercise. My grandfather walked many miles each day to work on a farm. He didn't have a car to take him to the grocery store. He had to work hard physically for his family's food.

Now, exercise is not a given. If we want to stay healthy, we need to make a daily effort to move vigorously. Join fitness classes at your gym, rec center, or swimming pool.

5) Medicine keeps us alive longer. Advances in sanitation, surgery, antibiotics, and medical care may keep you alive longer.

When you get old and sick, your kids won't leave you out in the wilderness to die, as was the solution to aging in times past. It is more likely that you will spend your last decades deaf, blind, mindless, and immobile in an overheated nursing home. You will be medicated, diapered, catheterized, spoon-fed, and finally intravenously fed until you finally somehow manage to die. It won't be easy to die, as the nursing home will be motivated to keep you alive in order to get paid. If you don't have a living will, your doctor is obligated to prolong your life at all costs.

This depressing picture doesn't have to happen. You can make changes now to prevent the inevitable hormone imbalance that accompanies aging, and in many cases is being experienced by young men also.

You don't have to get any of the diseases that are often inherited. Even though your genes may be programmed to cause disease and death, you can prevent this programming from playing out.

When it finally begins to dawn on a man that he is becoming old, he may wonder how to slow down or reverse the aging process. None of us can completely reverse aging. But we can modify and reverse many aspects of aging.

Testosterone is directly influenced by what you eat and the amount of exercise that you get.

A research team studied men who didn't exercise and ate the standard American diet. They rechecked them after they exercised for 150 minutes weekly and ate a diet with reduced fat and calories.[79] These men did not take supplemental testosterone.

Their testosterone went up just by exercising and improving their diets! Why? Their testosterone went up partially because the exercise and dietary changes improved their insulin and adrenal problems. None of the other hormones can be balanced until insulin is somewhat controlled and cortisol (that important adrenal stress hormone) levels are somewhat normalized. Insulin and adrenal problems are primarily lifestyle issues. Improve your lifestyle habits and your insulin and adrenals will get better. When insulin and adrenals improve, so will the other hormones.

Begin improving your lifestyle in order to optimize your hormones. Three major lifestyle factors are diet, exercise, and sleep. Other things that you can do to improve your lifestyle are to quit smoking, quit using recreational drugs, reduce the amount of toxicity you are taking in, reduce your exposure to toxic substances, and remove the toxins that are already in your body. To learn more about how to do these things, be sure to read our detailed guide, "Secrets to Lose Toxic Belly Fat!"[80]

Improve your diet.

Insulin is a hormone that often goes too high. As insulin rises, men get fat and find it extremely difficult to lose the fat.

Eating too many carbohydrates causes too much insulin, which causes the body to become insulin-resistant. This results in diabetes and metabolic syndrome (pre-diabetes).

An insulin-resistant man turns more of his testosterone into estrogen. It is a nasty, vicious cycle. This whole process creates fat. The fat makes even more insulin and estrogen, producing even more fat.

Control your carb intake and eat plenty of proteins, vegetables, and good fats. Eating this way helps you to overcome insulin resistance. Eating this way balances the two hormones that control your blood sugar. These two hormones are insulin and glucagon. Let's see how this works.

Insulin is released in response to carbohydrates. Prolonged, excessive carbohydrate intake produces excessive insulin. Prolonged excessive insulin produces insulin resistance. Insulin resistance makes you fat because it prevents stored body fat from being released. If there is excessive insulin, more food will be stored as fat. This is why we want to eat less of foods that increase insulin. That means you should always eat fat and protein with carbohydrate.

Glucagon is released in response to protein and low blood sugar. Glucagon causes fat loss. Glucagon opens up fat cells so that fat can be released and burned. If there is relatively more glucagon and less insulin, more food will be used as building materials or fuel. This means that we need to eat plenty of protein to balance the carbs that we eat.

Neither insulin nor glucagon is released in response to non-starchy vegetables and healthy fats. If fats or non-starchy vegetables are eaten, it won't affect either insulin or glucagon. Eating plenty of fats and non-starchy vegetables is important to give us the building blocks for hormones and the vitamins and minerals necessary for the proper functioning of our bodies.

To balance insulin and glucagon, eat proteins, good fats, non-starchy vegetables, and a moderate amount of low-glycemic carbohydrates together in the same meal. When carbohydrates are eaten without protein or fat, the insulin level goes too high as compared to glucagon, and the food is stored as fat. Include the good fats, non-starchy vegetables, and just the right amount of carbohydrate for the energy that you will burn off.

It is difficult to overeat when eating proteins and fat. CCK (cholecystokinin) is a hormone secreted from the intestinal walls in response to proteins and fats. CCK causes the gallbladder to contract and to secrete bile to absorb fats. CCK goes to the brain and lets it know that the body is being fed.

Too much CCK causes nausea. CCK makes it difficult to overeat when you eat proteins and fats. Digestion of carbohydrates does not cause CCK production.

When eating carbohydrates alone, there is no feeling of satiety until the carbohydrates are converted in the liver to glucose which goes to the brain and signals satiety. This takes about twenty minutes and allows you to overeat carbohydrates easily.

Eating the proteins and fats on your plate first will help you to avoid overeating. This will get that CCK hormone going to your brain.

Foods to decrease glucose and insulin:

- **Onions** lower glucose by competing with insulin, increasing insulin activity.
- **Brewer's yeast** is high in chromium which helps insulin bind to the cell receptors.
- **Cinnamon** may act as an insulin substitute and reduces blood sugar 20 to 30 percent.
- **Olive oil** improves blood sugar control while lowering triglycerides.

- **Beans, legumes, and nuts** have fiber which improves glucose tolerance and insulin sensitivity.
- **Mangoes** have a low glycemic index, high fiber, and high enzymes.

Balance proteins, low-glycemic carbs, and good fats. This way of eating balances your insulin levels and heals your metabolism.

When you first begin to eat this way, you may actually gain weight for a while because you are eating the building blocks for health. Do not be discouraged.

If you continue on with this healthy way of eating, your metabolism will finally be able to heal. After a period of time, you will notice that you are losing weight, as well as noticing improvement of all of your health problems.

When you get your insulin and glucose levels balanced, you will have more willpower. Your brain won't urge you to eat so often. It will become easier to eat correctly, to exercise, and to do things that are good for you that you couldn't do before.

Start exercising.

Motivation is tough, but just do it. For many people, it is tough to get going with an exercise program. They go to the doctor and expect a pill to take care of their weight and health problems. But no pill can take the place of physical activity. You just have to do it.

If you don't have the willpower to get going with an exercise program, find someone to exercise with. If you have a friend who will walk with you, then get together and always exercise at a certain time of each day. Get a dog. You have to walk the dog. Join a gym and get a personal trainer to design a program for you. Get a work-out partner to share in the fun. Go to exercise classes.

Years ago, people didn't have to worry about finding the time and motivation to exercise. Exercise was a part of everyday life. Now we have cars that take us to the supermarket. We sit in front of our computers and televisions. Our technological marvels make life so easy. But if we want to enjoy health, we must make a daily effort to exercise and eat properly. Before you go to the doctor for a pill to take care of your ills, exercise and eat properly. If everyone did this, we would see a reversal in most of the chronic diseases that we see today.

The bottom line on exercise is to do it and keep doing it for the rest of your life. The American College of Sports Medicine (ACSM) sums it up, "Emphasis should be placed on factors that result in permanent lifestyle change and encourage a lifetime of physical activity."[81]

The ACSM further states, "A well-rounded training program, including aerobic and resistance training and flexibility exercises, is recommended." A good work-out starts with a warm-up, then strength training, some endurance training, some sprinting, and some flexibility exercises at the end when your muscles are loose. There you have it.

But don't overdo. Excessive exercise can cause weight gain by harming your adrenals. It will cause too much cortisol (a stress hormone) to be produced. The cortisol causes fat to be stored,[82] pushing your adrenals into adrenal fatigue or exhaustion.

Excessive exercise also produces free radicals which cause inflammation. Don't exercise to exhaustion. Leave the gym when you still feel like you could exercise at least for the same amount of time that you already worked out. Don't forget to take antioxidants to handle free radical production.

When just beginning an exercise program, start with walking if you can. Can you walk? If the answer is yes, do it. Build up to an hour or more of walking each day.

If you are really sick and walking is a problem, start with a 5-15 minute walk (two and a half to seven minutes out and two and a half to seven minutes back). Then add a minute a week. The key is to do it every day, no matter what.

Don't just play your worry tapes while walking. Calm your mind and turn your walking into meditation, by saying the words, "Be here now." Practice being present in the moment.

If you walk for a half hour three times a day, you will actually burn more calories than you would if you walk for an hour and a half once a day. When you bump up your metabolism more frequently, it stays up so that you burn more calories even when you aren't exercising.

If you can't walk, find something you can do like riding a stationary bike. If you have knee/leg pain that limits walking, exercise in water. Join a gym and go. Just do it.

Forget about the amount of weight you need to lose. First concentrate on getting healthier. When you can burn 3000 calories a week at a moderately-intense level of activity (not working out all that hard) you will see improvement in every health-care marker. This includes triglycerides, blood pressure, body composition, HDL, and blood glucose tolerance. It is possible to cure type 2 diabetes, if caught early. Exercise and diet are essential to cure type 2 diabetes.[83] Without diet and exercise, nothing else works.

You will see improvement, even after the very first exercise session.[84] You will continue to improve with every exercise session. You will be able to return to the natural state of health that your body was designed for. You will sleep better. Disease will melt away as you keep at it. Your sex life will improve. There is no drug that can do what exercise will do.

Exercise which targets the burning of belly fat is important. Compared to fat found in the upper legs and buttocks, visceral fat (belly fat) is much more strongly linked to cardiovascular disease and diabetes.[85] Certainly any aerobic exercise will help you lose the belly fat. But it is also important to add in specific abdominal exercises such as Pilates and other core exercise routines to lose the dangerous abdominal fat.

Get plenty of quality sleep.

Getting plenty of undisturbed, deep sleep is critical for optimal hormones. If you wake up in the middle of the night and can't get back to sleep, or you have trouble falling asleep, your hormones will be imbalanced, or your sleep problem is the result of hormonal imbalance.

Do everything you can to minimize the stress in your life. Analyze your life and determine what is causing your stress. Then do what you can to eliminate or minimize the stress. Especially, change your attitude.

Practice good sleep hygiene. Stop watching violent or activating movies on TV, especially right before bed. At a set time every evening, turn the lights down low and read or enjoy pleasant conversation. Listen to soft music. Wind down. Taking supplemental calcium and magnesium at bedtime helps sleep. Don't forget your melatonin. A time-released version will take you through the night.

Aim to get as much sleep as you need. You may have to go to bed early to achieve this goal. If you wake up and can't get back to sleep, take some more magnesium. Many people find meditation helpful to help them go back to sleep again. Sometimes a coffee enema may help you get back to sleep. The coffee enema causes your liver to dump its toxins into the intestines where they can be removed. This calms you down so that you can sleep again.

What you don't want to do is stay up late or get up in the middle of the night and work on the computer. Any light coming into your eyes tells your body that it is time to wake up. Your objective is to go to sleep and stay asleep during the night.

Cleansing and detoxification.

We all live in a polluted and toxic world. The first step in cleansing is to eliminate incoming toxins. Avoid processed food and drinks. Avoid GMO foods. Eat organic fruits and vegetables. A healthy diet, high in live food with natural vegetable fibers is necessary for intestinal health. Our goal is to gradually eliminate the toxins through the eliminative organs, like the skin, the intestines, and the kidneys.

The large intestine is the first and foremost way that the body cleans out the poisons. If there is good and effective intestinal cleansing, with lots of natural fiber, the body can cleanse itself. If not, the toxins will diffuse back into the blood.

Adding natural fibers and bentonite clay are very effective. Activated charcoal and bentonite clay bind toxins until they can be excreted.

More effective intestinal cleansers, like coffee enemas, can be used for more toxic conditions. Coffee enemas are used in many treatment programs for serious diseases, such as cancer and diabetes. Colonics are popular and effective, but expensive, requiring high levels of sanitation at the colonic facility. Home enemas are cheaper and more convenient.

Effective functioning of the liver detoxification process is the second avenue of excretion. These detoxification cycles require sulfur-containing amino acids, minerals, especially selenium, and vitamins to function. The loss of any one of these will block the function of the entire detox cycle.

Sweating through the skin is the third avenue of excretion of toxins. Saunas and far-infrared saunas are great tools of detoxification. Hard exercise that makes you sweat is good, too.

Last is mobilizing toxins from the matrix stores. The problem is that most of us have so much toxicity stored in the matrix that it is dangerous to mobilize them too quickly.

It is dangerous to drastically reduce your food intake by dieting or fasting when you have a lot of toxicity in your body. Fasting has been advocated for centuries for spiritual and physical cleansing. But it may be risky. One risk of fasting is that it can lead to thyroid dysfunction. If done incorrectly, fasting can be hazardous or even fatal.

When you fast, the body will start to dump the toxins that are stored in the matrix. You need to pace yourself, so that you do not overwhelm the eliminative organs. Otherwise, the poisons may damage your vital organs. Consulting experts about how to fast is essential.

If you cannot metabolize the toxins in the liver and then excrete them through the intestines, the toxins will end up in your brain and kidneys. Electrolyte imbalances may occur and can be fatal.

If you fast, do it wisely and under supervision until you understand it well. Short fruit fasts are the easiest and safest way to start. A good short fruit fast would be to eat only apples for a day or two.

If you get into juice fasts, enemas are necessary. If you have weakened adrenals, blood sugar issues, or thyroid problems, do not fast. Detoxification with homeopathics is effective, safe, and easy.

Rolfing and other deep tissue manipulations mobilize toxins. To maximize the healing benefits of these therapies, attend to cleansing procedures after deep tissue manipulations.

Always start slowly. Be gentle to your body. If you have a proven toxic burden, it may take the rest of your life to cleanse it out. Cleansing and detoxification are lifestyle practices for many of us who suffer from intoxication. A lifetime of cleansing allows those of us with serious toxicity to live long, healthy lives.

For detailed instructions on cleansing, please refer to our book, "Secrets to Lose Toxic Belly Fat!" This is book six in the Bioidentical Hormones series.[86]

Coffee enemas are safe and easy. They are an effective method of helping you to attain a superior state of health, because they cause your body to dump toxicity.

Don't rule out this important anti-aging tool, just because of squeamishness. Try using coffee enemas for a few weeks before you make any judgment about their worthiness. Coffee enemas are a most important liver detoxification tool. Coffee enemas are major components of many treatment programs for degenerative diseases such as arthritis and diabetes. Take coffee enemas regularly to cleanse the liver and intestines of toxicity.

Coffee enemas became established into medicine when Dr. Max Gerson began using them to treat cancer patients in the 1930's.[87] Substances in coffee detoxify carcinogens by neutralizing free radicals. Most proponents believe that the major value of the coffee enema is that a coffee enema retained for fifteen minutes will cause the liver to dump its toxic load. The coffee is absorbed directly into the bloodstream, where it is carried to the liver and gall bladder. The coffee stimulates the liver and gallbladder to dump toxins into the lumen of the intestines, where they can be excreted from the body. Taking organic chlorella an hour before the coffee enema will help bind toxic substances in the bile,[88] [89] [90] so that they can be eliminated.

When doing any kind of enema, it is important to minimize the risks involved by using liquid that is no warmer than room temperature, sterilizing equipment, and never sharing equipment. Never use tap water that has not been boiled and filtered. The intestines may easily be contaminated with bacteria, viruses, and parasites from water. Lube the tip to avoid tearing anal tissue.

To take a coffee enema, begin by using only a small amount of coffee (a half teaspoon) in a 12-cup coffee maker. You may work up to three tablespoons of coffee if it doesn't irritate the intestines and isn't too stimulating. Let the coffee cool to room temperature. Then pour it into a gravity-drainage enema bag that you can get at the drug store. Prop up the hips with towel-covered pillows placed next to the toilet. Lube the tip with A&D ointment or oil and gently insert into the anus. Control the flow with the valve. Allow the liquid to run in slowly, a cup at a time, until you feel full. To move the enema through the colon, you may start on the left side, turn to your back, and then go to the right side, then back on the left, all the while massaging your belly to loosen waste. You are loosening the waste up the right side of the belly, across the top, and down the left side. Try to hold the mixture as long as possible. Some people will only be able to manage a few seconds. Others may be able to hold it longer. Fifteen minutes is ideal. Don't worry if you can't hold it for a long time. Don't worry if nothing comes out. In this case, you are dehydrated and have absorbed the liquid. You may follow the coffee mixture with plain water to rinse out the coffee. A second enema four to six hours after the first can greatly speed the exit of toxins pulled out during the first enema. Other important cleansing methods include saunas, infrared saunas, short fasts, and cleansing of chemicals and heavy metals through chelation and other cleanses. For a thorough discussion of cleansing toxicity from your body, thoroughly read, "Secrets to Lose Toxic Belly Fat!" [91]

CHAPTER 12. CONTRAINDICATIONS TO T THERAPY.

YOU SHOULD NOT BEGIN TESTOSTERONE THERAPY IF YOU HAVE ANY OF THE CONDITIONS LISTED IN THIS SECTION. These conditions are so risky that the potential benefit cannot outweigh the potential risk of testosterone therapy.

Desire to remain fertile.

Your testicles will shrink when you supplement with testosterone. Testosterone decreases LH and FSH which causes a decrease in testicular volume.

Testosterone decreases sperm because of testicular atrophy, decreasing fertility. If you use testosterone, you may become unable to father children.

Testosterone therapy will so greatly impair fertility that it cannot be done if maintaining fertility is important to you. Testosterone therapy inhibits gonadotropin release from the pituitary. When the gonadotropins, LH and FSH decrease, the testes atrophy.

This results in reduced sperm production. This is an effect that increases with the dosage of testosterone and duration of treatment.

It is reversible in short-term testosterone therapy, but irreversible atrophy occurs with prolonged treatment. If you want to remain fertile, hCG and Clomiphene (Clomid) are safe and effective alternatives.

HCG and Clomid are treatment options to increase testosterone without adversely effecting testes function and sperm production. HCG has more of an action like LH and is less effective for fertility. Clomiphene has FSH and LH action and is used in male infertility to increase sperm production.

Lower urinary tract obstruction.

Consultation with a urologist is essential for patients with lower urinary tract obstruction. In a case-by-case basis and approval by your urologist, testosterone therapy might be considered. If the potential benefit is considered to greatly outweigh the potential risk, testosterone therapy might be conducted very slowly with intense follow up.

Untreated obstructive sleep apnea (OSA):

Testosterone therapy has been shown to worsen sleep-disordered breathing among patients with severe obstructive sleep apnea,[92] which is a risk for atherosclerosis.[93] Once the obstructive sleep apnea is treated, testosterone therapy may be considered on a case-by-case basis. There is an association of obstructive sleep apnea with increased visceral adiposity and low testosterone values. Obstructive sleep apnea is associated with visceral obesity, insulin resistance, hypertension, and cardiovascular disease. The presence of low testosterone complicates obstructive sleep apnea because of the cardiovascular risk factors associated with low testosterone. Some studies have shown that testosterone can be associated with exacerbations of obstructive sleep apnea. Because of this, patients (especially elderly patients) should not be started on testosterone therapy until the obstructive sleep apnea is adequately treated. Studies have shown no significant difference in the frequency of obstructive sleep apnea from testosterone therapy.[94][95] Even though several small studies have shown benefit to patients with obstructive sleep apnea, [96][97][98] caution must be taken when using testosterone therapy in these patients.

Prostate or breast cancer:

Again in selected cases and under the strict supervision of all treating physicians, if greater potential benefit exists, careful testosterone therapy may be considered. Otherwise, testosterone therapy should not be used.

CHAPTER 13. RELATIVE CONTRAINDICATIONS.

CONDITIONS THAT HAVE SIGNIFICANTLY INCREASED RISK ARE CALLED RELATIVE CONTRAINDICATIONS. In these instances, testosterone therapy should only be considered when the potential benefits are great. Very close supervision is required.

Poorly controlled heart failure.

Once the patient is stabilized and maximal control of the heart failure is obtained, very slow administration of testosterone therapy may only be considered in selected cases.

With unstable angina or congestive heart failure, start treatment carefully and responsibly. Start with very low dosages and increase slowly. Abrupt initiation of treatment can stress the heart and precipitate increased congestive heart failure or a heart attack.

Men with a high risk of prostate cancer.

Individuals with high risk for prostate cancer should be evaluated by a urologist prior to the initiation of testosterone therapy and very careful monitoring of prostate exam and PSA levels while on testosterone therapy.

Concerns for the safety of testosterone therapy and the prostate have been raised by studies showing metastatic prostate cancer after the initiation of testosterone therapy.[99][100][101] This has led to the consideration of patients at high risk for prostate cancer as a relative contraindication for testosterone therapy.

Most studies have not revealed an increased risk of prostate cancer in testosterone therapy. [102][103][104][105] One meta-analysis found no significantly increased incidence of prostate cancer with testosterone therapy.[106] Other small studies have found no increased prostate cancer in men treated for prostate cancer.[107][108][109]

Elevated estrogen.

Testosterone is aromatized into estrogen by fat cells, so **patients with visceral obesity are at a much greater risk** for abnormal estrogen elevations than non-obese patients. This produces feminine side effects with gynecomastia (man-boobs) and increased obesity.

The prostate can be adversely affected by the increased estrogen. 16-OH-estrone is created by pathologic estrogen metabolism. This harmful estrogen metabolite is especially irritating to the prostate tissue. 16-OH-estrone is associated with increased cancer especially in breast and prostate.   Hypogonadal men who are obese not only further lower their testosterone by this aromatization in fat cells, but also create estrogenic effects that counter the effects of their already-low testosterone.

Elevated red blood cell count.

Men with hypogonadism have lower hemoglobin levels. Testosterone therapy has been shown to restore the hemoglobin levels of older men.   The hematocrit is the percentage of your blood that is made up of red blood cells. It goes up with testosterone therapy.

Testosterone may excessively increase red blood cells (erythrocytosis). This is more likely with injections. Men with COPD, smokers, and those with sleep apnea are more at risk. You can solve this problem by giving blood or discarding it at hematocrit greater than 55 to get rid of excess iron. The increase in the hematocrit and hemoglobin associated with testosterone therapy can excessively increase the blood viscosity (thickness), predisposing patients to abnormal clotting and an associated increase in cardiovascular disease. This predisposes patients with hematocrits greater than 54 to the risk of thrombotic complications including stroke, DVT (leg clots), and heart attacks.

Careful monitoring of the hematocrit in testosterone therapy is required to safely administer testosterone therapy. If you have a hematocrit that is greater than 50%, testosterone therapy should be considered only with careful follow up and the drawing-off of excess blood on a case-by-case basis.   If the hematocrit goes above 54%, getting rid of excess blood would be necessary to lower the hematocrit.

In many of the studies that show increased cardiovascular complications during testosterone replacement, unsafe increases in the hematocrit could have been the underlying problem.   Because they did not monitor the hematocrit, we will never know.

Deep venous thrombosis (clots in veins).

In 2014, the FDA placed a new warning on testosterone therapy regarding venous thrombosis and testosterone therapy. They noted that in addition to the known risk of thrombotic events as a result of polycythemia from testosterone therapy, they had received reports of venous thrombosis during testosterone therapy unrelated to polycythemia.

One of the reasons for this new concern was a study done by Glueck et al. and published in 2014.[110] They looked at testosterone therapy in 596 men with deep venous thrombosis/pulmonary embolism (DVT-PE).   Seven episodes of DVT-PE occurred in men who were on testosterone therapy and had abnormalities in the clotting mechanism prior to the testosterone therapy.

Dr. Glueck recommends that certain clotting disorders should be ruled out before testosterone therapy. This would involve four blood tests at a cost of around $800. He further notes that elevated estrogen may be the agent causing the increased clotting in these patients. However, anastrozole is prothrombotic in these patients, so there is concern for the use of aromatase inhibitors in these patients. Until this concern is thoroughly understood, patients on testosterone therapy should be aware of increased thrombotic risk and contact their physician if they have lower extremity edema with or without shortness of breath.

CHAPTER 14. RAISE TESTOSTERONE WITHOUT DRUGS.

Men may be able to bring their testosterone levels up with lifestyle, diet, and supplements alone. It depends on the reason for the low testosterone.

Testosterone levels drop when there is toxicity in the body. The drop in testosterone levels in all men everywhere may be caused by the increase in toxicity coming in from environmental pollution and also from bad lifestyle choices, such as smoking, drinking, and drug use.

Try these methods to boost testosterone.

- Winning.
- Improve adrenals.
- Improve sick metabolism--increase protein, eliminate alcohol, quit smoking.
- Decrease calories. Lose weight, especially belly fat.[111]
- Exercise, especially strength training.
- Supplement with lots of zinc, which is needed to metabolize testosterone.
- Avoid increased estrogen and get rid of xenoestrogens.
- Improve estrogen metabolism.
- Treat hypothyroidism.
- Treat methyl-mercury toxicity.

Boost testosterone with herbs.

Herbs are especially effective in treating suboptimal low testosterone. Natural herbal alternatives to increase testosterone and support the treatment of hypogonadism, erectile dysfunction, and loss of libido:

Tribulus terrestris: This herb from the puncture vine, also called goathead and many other names, has been used for centuries in China and India to enhance testosterone and virility.

In Ayurvedic medicine and Traditional Chinese Medicine it is used to treat diseases of the liver and kidney, as an aphrodisiac, and as an anabolic stimulant to increase muscle. It reportedly increases testosterone in men and women by increasing LH levels which stimulates increased testosterone in men and increased testosterone and estrogen in women. However, Tribulus failed to raise testosterone in three controlled studies and failed to increase strength in a fourth.

It was popularized by Jeffrey Peterman, a champion body builder in the '70s and is still used by some body builders as post-cycle therapy. The belief is that testosterone will be increased after an anabolic cycle of hormones.

The active chemical, protodioscin, is related to DHEA, the direct precursor for testosterone. It is thought that protodioscin corrects infertility, increases libido, and improves erectile dysfunction. It has been shown to increase low sperm counts. Protodioscin improves sexual desire and helps erections through converting to DHEA.[112]

As with DHEA supplementation, patients with hormone-related conditions and pregnant/nursing women should not use it. It has an excellent safety profile. If you feel a stomach ache with it, this would be alleviated by taking it with food. It can have a negative effect on your sleep and some research has suggested that it can increase prostate size.

Horny Goat weed (Epimedium): This Chinese herb is well-known for its ability to increase testosterone and improve libido. According to legend, a Chinese goat herder noticed increased sexual activity in his goats after eating this herb.

The active chemical is icariin, which is a phosphodiesterase type 5 inhibitor (PDE5 inhibitor) like Viagra. Icariin also enhances nitric oxide secretion which relaxes smooth muscle. Nitric oxide is essential for erection. This relaxation of tension deep in the smooth muscles of the internal tissues produces a broad range of healing benefits.

It is used extensively in Traditional Chinese Medicine to relieve fatigue in the mind and body, treat osteoporosis, and for sexual dysfunction. It stimulates osteoblastic bone activity and there are several medicinal products for osteoporosis with icariin.[113] Structurally-modified icariin has been shown to be a more specific inhibitor of PDE-5 than Viagra.

Bulbine natalensis: This South African herb has been traditionally used for many years by the indigenous peoples for its aphrodisiac qualities and its reported ability to increase testosterone levels. Three studies in rats have shown a large increase in testosterone (346%) as well as increases in LH, FSH, progesterone, with no effect on prolactin, and a decrease in estrogen.[114 115 116]

However the rat studies showed consistent pathological damage to the liver and kidneys. Lipid values were also significantly worsened.   These adverse effects occurred at the dosage required to increase testosterone.

Bulbine natalensis has aphrodisiac qualities. Testicular size is increased, but prostate and other male tissues were unaffected in the rat studies.

Macuna pruriens: High levels of L-dopa in the seeds of this herb are converted to dopamine, which not only increases testosterone and HGH (growth hormone) levels but most effectively decreases elevated prolactin levels.

Macuna's sexual benefits have been best studied in infertile males. Macuna increased testosterone, LH, sperm counts, and dopamine in several double blind studies of infertile males. The increased testosterone is thought to be because of the suppressive effects of dopamine on prolactin.[117]

In Parkinson's disease large doses have been shown to be as effective as pure L-dopa/carbidopa, but long-term efficacy and safety are unknown.[118] It should not be used in pregnancy or by schizophrenics.

Tongkat ali (Eurycoma longifolia): This Malaysian herb has been used for thousands of years and has glycopeptides that are reported to raise free testosterone levels, reduce sex hormone binding globulins, and increase muscle growth. It enhances sperm count and sperm motility and muscle growth.[119] The government of Malaysia and Massachusetts Institute of

Technology hold patents on the water extract of Eurycoma for sexual dysfunction and male infertility.

Suma: This herb, also called Brazilian ginseng, is in the root of the suma vine in South America. It is used for symptoms of andropause and sexual dysfunction. The active chemical is thought to be ecdysterone, which is reported to support testosterone in men and stimulate sexual performance.

Maca: This South American herb, also called Peruvian ginseng, has been popular for five thousand years as an aphrodisiac. Incan imperial warriors ate large amounts of maca prior to battle and after a city was conquered. The sexual virility of the warriors was legendary.

The aphrodisiac effect of maca is reportedly from the chemical p-methoxybenzyl isothiodyanate.[120] Glucosinolates are an important part of the aphrodisiac and energizing effects, restoring vitality and balancing the nervous system. Studies have shown improvement in sperm and semen.[121]

Avena sativa (Oats, oatstraw): This herb is thought to stimulate LH and therefore testosterone. Oat extract is soothing to the brain and nervous system, and increases sexual desire and performance in both men and women. This is where the saying "sowing your wild oats" comes from. It is reported to have beneficial effects on sexual response, libido, and orgasm.[122] Its benefit is thought to be from enhanced blood flow.

Chrysin: Chrysin is an extract from the plant, Passiflora coerulea, that has been shown in vitro (in test tubes) to be a natural inhibitor of aromatase, which converts testosterone to estrogen. It therefore would be expected to not only raise testosterone, but also to lower estrogen. This would be of special benefit in estrogen-dominant men (mainly men who are overweight), since aromatase is found in fat tissue. However, in vivo studies (in live animals and humans) show no effect on estrogen levels. Follow-up studies determined that cell membranes effectively block chrysin from entering the cells and having any effect.[123]

Muira puama (ptychopetalum): is called "potency wood" in its native Amazon rain forest. As its name implies, it is used by the indigenous people to enhance sexual performance.   A study done at the Institute of Sexology in Paris found that 62% of men reported an increase in sex drive and 51% an increased ability to produce an erection.[124] A UCLA School of Medicine study showed improvement in erectile function and sex drive. It increases blood flow to pelvic organs and can slightly increase blood pressure.[125]

Damiana (Turnera Aphrodisiaca): Damiana leaves have been used by Mayan Indians and Mexicans to boost the sexual potency of both men and women for centuries. It has also been used as a general tonic and held to be efficacious in mild depression. It increases energy levels, which helps restore libido and acts as an aphrodisiac in both men and women. It stimulates increased blood flow and oxygen to genital tissues. Exactly how it works is not known.

Yohimbine hydrochloride: is found in the bark of an African tree. It is a stimulant with aphrodisiac and mild monoamine oxidase inhibitor effects. Inhibitors of monoamine oxidase, a class of antidepressants, normally have severe reactions with the amino acid tyramine, but this does not occur with yohimbine.

It is available as a prescription drug and the National Institutes of Health states it is an effective treatment of male impotence.[126]   It has also been shown to be effective as a treatment for orgasmic dysfunction in men[127] and low sexual desire in women. Yohimbine is used to counteract the side effects of the SSRI class of antidepressants, especially the sexual side effects and dry mouth, and as a treatment for xerostomia (dry mouth).

It can cause dangerous side effects and the range between the effective dose and the dangerous dose is small.   It causes increased blood pressure in small amounts and dangerous decreases in large doses. It can cause a prolonged erection (priapism), which can be a medical emergency. Panic, hallucinations, and paralysis can occur as well. It should not be used by anyone with liver, kidney, or heart disease, or a psychological disorder.

Catuaba: The bark of this South American tree is used in the traditional medicine of Brazil for its aphrodisiac and central nervous system stimulant effects. It is widely sold as an aphrodisiac and remedy for erectile dysfunction. The sexual benefits are thought to come from the alkaloids (catuabine A, B, and C). Although no large- scale scientific studies have confirmed its benefits, it is thought to increase blood flow to the penis, creating a stronger erection that lasts longer. It may also increase the brain's sensitivity to dopamine which creates an enhanced sexual experience.

Ginkgo biloba: This herb from the maidenhair tree has been used in Traditional Chinese Medicine for over 4,000 years. The flavonoids have a strong antioxidant effect and are prized in anti-aging medicine. The ginkgogolides and bilobalides have antiplatelet effects to decrease clotting and also improve circulation. In traditional Chinese medicine, ginkgo is used for its anti-aging effect, treatment of tinnitus (ringing in the ears), cerebral disorders of dementia and Parkinson's, treatment of asthma and respiratory disorders, and for its aphrodisiac effect. It is best known as an enhancer of memory, probably through its effect of increasing circulation to the brain.

Increased blood flow to the pelvic organs is thought to be a part of its benefit in sexual function. One well-known study showed close to 80% success in treating erectile impotence.[128] Another study found it to be 84% effective in the treatment of the sexual side effects of the SSRI antidepressants, and benefits in all phases of the sexual cycle – desire, erection and lubrication, orgasm, and afterglow. This study was initiated because geriatric patients taking gingko for memory enhancement noted improved erections.[129]   However, two other studies did not show significant benefits.

Gingko's benefit to sexual function is enhanced when it is combined with ginseng, tribulus, or maca. Improving sexual function takes at least 6-8 weeks. It is contraindicated in patients on anticoagulants, pre-surgery, pregnancy, and epileptics.

Ginseng: Ginseng has been used for over 4,000 years in Traditional Chinese Medicine for its effect as a tonic for the male, its ability to improve vitality, its anti-fatigue effects, type 2 diabetes treatment, and its action as an aphrodisiac and cure for sexual dysfunction in men. The therapeutic benefits are from the ginsenosides in the root.

The red Panax ginseng results from the root being steamed and then dried. It is a promoter of yang energy.

White ginseng is Panax quinquefolius, also known as American ginseng. It is considered a promoter of yin energy. Panax ginseng is safe even in large amounts, but overdoses can precipitate irritability, increased blood pressure, and bleeding.

Ginseng is contraindicated in hypertension, combined with other stimulants, and in patients with heart problems.

Fenugreek (trigonella foenum-graecum): Fenugreek is best known as a spice used in curry and other spicy dishes. It has traditionally been used for augmenting breast milk, increasing glucose utilization, heartburn and GI disturbances, and improving lipid profiles.

Use with caution! Because of its effectiveness in augmenting breast milk production there is concern that fenugreek may increase prolactin secretion.

Fenugreek also has the reputation of increasing libido, improving athletic performance, and increasing testosterone. Fenugreek has aromatase and 5-alpha reductase enzymes. Many studies have shown no testosterone improvement although some studies have shown the opposite. One study evaluated the effects of fenugreek on athletic performance in thirty men. They found increased performance in weight lifting, reduced body fat and increased testosterone levels.[130] It is probable that it does increase testosterone by its 5-alpha reductase activity to decrease the conversion of testosterone to DHT. Another study found improved libido and sexual energy in sixty men.[131]

Boost testosterone with supplements.

Natural supplements to increase testosterone:

Zinc: Zinc is required to make testosterone. Symptoms of zinc deficiency include delayed sexual development, hypogonadism, impotency, and decreased sexual desire. When zinc deficiency is present, zinc is dramatic in its ability to increase testosterone.[132] The highest levels of zinc in the body are in the prostate and sperm.

Vitamin A: This important vitamin is important in the function of the testes. Higher vitamin A levels in the testes increase testosterone secretion and a variety of powerful cellular growth factors.

Arginine: This nonessential amino acid is found in a wide variety of foods. It has been shown to increase HGH (growth hormone) secretion and is the direct precursor for nitric oxide, so important in the healthy function of the blood vessels. It decreases the healing time for damaged tissue and decreases the blood pressure in some patients with hypertension. Taken with pycnogenol, it improves erectile dysfunction,[133] or taken with glutamic acid and yohimbine, it also improves erectile dysfunction.[134]

Citrulline: This amino acid can be converted into arginine and therefore has been used to lower blood pressure and to treat mild erectile dysfunction.[135]

D-aspartic acid: This amino acid is relatively new and not much is known about its benefits or its long-term risks. One study in 2009 found it increased testosterone and LH. It increased aromatization in several animal studies, so there is concern about this also.

Phosphatidylserine: This is the most commonly used supplement to lower cortisol. It helps lower the night time elevations that disturb sleep and helps daytime control in stage 1 adrenal dysfunction. Anything that normalizes and lowers cortisol also benefits testosterone levels.

Boron: Boron is an ultratrace mineral and is essential for plants and animals. Such small amounts are needed that no deficiency state is known.

Disodium tetraborate, better known as borax, is commonly used to kill ants and cockroaches.

Its value in raising testosterone was established in 2011 in a landmark study of boron supplementation and its effect on testosterone and inflammatory cytokines.[136] Eight males ingested ten mg of boron daily for a week. The study found a 28% increase in free testosterone and a 39% decrease in estradiol! Even more impressive, the inflammatory cytokines, TNF alpha and IL6, significantly decreased with a decrease in the inflammatory marker, hsCRP. Boron is also known to decrease SHBG. Little is known of toxicity but there is concern for long-term consumption of boron.

Vitamin C: Vitamin C lowers cortisol in mega doses and has been shown to decrease the cortisol elevation after excessive exercise. Anything that lowers cortisol benefits testosterone. As an antioxidant and its efficiency in treating infectious disease, it also has the known benefit of producing healthy connective tissue.

Magnesium: Magnesium has been shown to increase testosterone when combined with exercise. Magnesium also has a multitude of other beneficial actions in the human body.

Astaxanthin and saw palmetto: The combination of these two has been shown in two studies to increase testosterone and decrease estradiol and DHT.[137] [138]

CHAPTER 15. BOOST TESTOSTERONE AND MAINTAIN FERTILITY.

Whenever you use testosterone, you do so at the risk of decreasing fertility. Once you begin to use supplemental testosterone, the testes will decrease their normal production of testosterone. Your fertility drops. You may not be able to father a child again.

When you use supplemental testosterone, the pituitary gland in the brain senses that you now have enough testosterone. The pituitary stops trying to stimulate the testes to produce testosterone.

Your testicles shrink a bit, because they are not being used to make testosterone. Your testicles stop producing as much sperm, and you may become infertile.

There are several little-known ways to use pharmaceutical hormones and drugs to raise testosterone while still maintaining fertility. Of course, if the testes cannot produce testosterone anymore, these methods will not work. You can either stimulate the production of gonadotropins (LH and FSH) with Clomiphene or you can give the gonadotropins (hCG, LH, or FSH). HCG is the only commonly used gonadotropin, because it is relatively inexpensive compared to the others. So we will only consider hCG and Clomiphene.

hCG (human Chorionic Gonadotropin) injections.

Testosterone levels may be increased in some men by using hCG (human Chorionic Gonadotropin) injections.[139] HCG is a hormone made by the placenta in pregnant women. HCG has very little FSH activity and primarily has LH activity.

HCG is useful when it is important to maintain fertility. Unlike using testosterone replacement methods, hCG can raise testosterone without lowering sperm count or losing testicular volume (shrinking testicles).[140] HCG is the primary option to treat low testosterone levels without stopping your own production of testosterone.

But hCG only works for men with low levels of LH. LH (luteinizing hormone) is a hormone that is secreted from the pituitary gland in the brain to stimulate the Leydig cells in the testes. HCG works because it acts like LH to stimulate the Leydig cells in the testes to produce testosterone.

If a man has low levels of LH, hCG use will stimulate his testes to produce more testosterone naturally. HCG use in men with low LH and FSH will also support increased sperm production.

LH can be measured with a blood or saliva test. Blood is preferable. To see if hCG might work for you to raise your testosterone levels by increasing production from your testes, you will need to get your LH levels tested. If LH is relatively low, maybe hCG will work, because the Leydig cells are still functioning.   You won't know until you try it and see if the testosterone levels go up.

In older men, low testosterone levels are often associated with high levels of LH. In older men, the Leydig cells in the testes stop responding to the LH.   The pituitary makes more and more LH in a futile attempt to get the Leydig cells to produce more testosterone. But the Leydig cells don't function as well anymore, no matter how much LH the pituitary sends out.

HCG won't work for men with high levels of LH. Because hCG works like LH to stimulate the Leydig cells in the testes to produce testosterone, hCG will not work in a man with high LH. If the LH isn't stimulating the testes to produce testosterone, neither will the hCG.

In low LH hypogonadism, the problem is in the brain. The reason for low testosterone may be caused from something like toxicity. If the Leydig cells are still functioning, as they are in most younger men, hCG may work to raise testosterone.

The cause of most low LH hypogonadism is unknown. Most patients do not suffer from the known causes--tumors or disorders that infiltrate the area of the pituitary, injury from chemotherapy or radiation, severe chronic diseases or malnutrition. In modern times, toxicity should be high on the list of causes, especially heavy metal and especially mercury. State-of-the-art medical testing for toxic chemicals and heavy metals is appropriate for all men with low LH disorders.

HCG will only work for a few years, though. Ultimately the hypogonadism will need testosterone replacement.

HCG is widely known for its use in weight loss. The dosage used to treat hypogonadism is approximately ten times the dosage used for the treatment of obesity. HCG can be used daily to achieve a blood level of testosterone that is steady. HCG is best delivered subcutaneously (under the skin). The package insert says intramuscular (into the muscle), but subcutaneous works well also. Subcutaneous administration is easier, doesn't hurt, and has delayed absorption. Your doctor would show you how to administer the hCG. HCG is an option that you can discuss with your physician if maintaining fertility is important to you. However, most primary-care physicians will not be aware of how to use hCG to treat men with low testosterone who also have low LH. Only anti-aging physicians will offer you this option.

Another option would be to combine both hCG and testosterone. This will help to somewhat avoid the side effects of testicular atrophy and lowered sperm count.[141] [142] Athletes who are sophisticated in the use of anabolic steroids use hCG for this reason. Consult your anti-aging doctor.

Clomiphene works so well that the NFL banned it.

Clomiphene will elevate testosterone similar to hCG. It is banned in the National Football League because of its ability to raise testosterone. Recently, an NFL player was suspended for use of clomiphene for four games.[143] Clomiphene is used for the diagnosis of hypogonadism and the treatment of infertility. Clomiphene (Clomid) is an often used female fertility drug and is often in the news because it often produces multiple births. It is also a useful male fertility drug as it stimulates sperm formation by its effect to increase FSH. It induces ovulation in the female by elevating LH and FSH levels by its action on the hypothalamus to block estrogen. Clomiphene is a drug that acts like a gonadotropin. It is a nonsteroidal estrogen antagonist at the hypothalamus and therefore stimulates the release of LH and FSH from the pituitary. Because of its stimulation of FSH, Clomiphene has a legitimate use in male infertility with low sperm counts and is still used for this.

CHAPTER 16. WHEN YOUR BODY CAN'T USE TESTOSTERONE.

Some men have plenty of testosterone, but it isn't in a form that they can use. Too much of their testosterone is bound up, so that it isn't available to be used when it is needed. Their test results show that they have a lot of total testosterone, but not much "bioavailable" testosterone.

Bioavailable testosterone is the testosterone that you can use. If you know the total and the free testosterone, then you can calculate the bioavailable testosterone. There is a free calculator for that on the internet.

Too much sex hormone-binding globulin (SHBG) drops your bioavailable testosterone. Sex hormone-binding globulin binds sex hormones and keeps them inactive until they are needed. As SHBG levels go up, more testosterone becomes bound up, so the bioavailable testosterone (usable) goes down.

If this is the case, taking supplemental testosterone may not solve your problem. Instead, you would have to lower the sex hormone-binding globulin and then retest for bioavailable testosterone.

Treatment of elevated SHBG levels is important when the free testosterone is significantly decreased.

- The first step is to treat any associated medical disorders or causes for elevated SHBG:
    - Elevated estrogen levels.
    - Elevated thyroid hormone levels.
    - Diseases of the liver (cirrhosis, and non-alcoholic fatty liver).
    - Severe malnutrition.
    - HIV infection.
    - Genetic conditions.
    - Aging.

- o Anticonvulsants.
- o Alcohol use.
- o Anti-hypertensives.
- o Sedatives.
- o Tranquilizers.

- **Boron is perhaps the best option,** as it has remarkable actions to decrease inflammation, as well as decrease SHBG and estradiol, while increasing free testosterone. Men taking 10 mg of disodium tetraborate (borax) had an increase in their free testosterone of 28% and a decrease of estradiol of 39%. Key inflammation chemicals (TNF-alpha and interleukin 6) decreased. (TNF-alpha is a key inflammatory cytokine involved in diabetes, heart disease, and arthritis.)[144]   Side effects or dangers from long-term boron use are unknown.

- Increase protein in the diet.

- Increase dietary fat.

- Increase omega-3 fish oils.

- Stinging nettle is proven to lower SHBG, but it lowers DHT as well, a necessary and important androgen. Since SHBG binds DHT more avidly than testosterone, it is a tricky balance between making less DHT and freeing up a bit more testosterone.

- DHEA lowers SHBG, but using DHEA can be unpredictable. It can raise testosterone, but it can unpredictably cause marked elevations of estradiol as well.

- Tongkat ali extract has been shown not only to lower SHBG but to raise free testosterone.[145]

- Vitamin D was found in one study to lower SHBG and to increase both free and total testosterone.[146]

- And finally, hormone replacement therapy lowers SHBG.

Develop a reasonable treatment plan, stick to it, and 2-4 months later check your SHBG levels and free testosterone.

CHAPTER 17. CAN YOU GET A PRESCRIPTION?

ALL DOCTORS SHOULD UNDERSTAND THE IMPORTANCE OF TREATING HYPOGONADISM. Nevertheless, there are some physicians who hold the philosophy that there is no such thing as hypogonadism. These doctors never write prescriptions for testosterone, no matter how low your levels may be.

If you are hypogonadal (testosterone below 300 ng/dl), it should not be difficult to get a prescription. Most physicians will write the prescription if you meet the strict criteria for hypogonadism. As physicians grow in their understanding of the devastating consequences of low testosterone in men, they are writing many more prescriptions for testosterone.[147]

But, if your testosterone level is low for you, but still above the lab reference value that represents hypogonadism, you will probably not get a prescription unless you are seeing an anti-aging doctor. Most physicians will not treat the sub-clinical or sub-optimal types of low testosterone.

Optimizing testosterone levels will be most effective if you also incorporate proper lifestyle, nutrition, nutritional supplements, dietary restrictions and exercise. Before writing a prescription, your doctor will take your medical history, give you a physical examination, and order tests. If you are deficient, your physician will monitor adverse side effects and adjust testosterone dosage based on your lab tests.

Find the right doctor.

IF A MAN IS DEFICIENT IN MALE SEX HORMONES, HE WILL BE TREATED BY MOST PHYSICIANS. A man can walk into almost any doctor's office and, if tests show an abnormally low level of testosterone, he can easily get a prescription for bioidentical testosterone (exactly like the testosterone his own body makes). Doctors are obligated to bring a man's sex hormone levels back up into the normal range when they are hypogonadal, because that is the standard of care. All knowledgeable doctors agree that low testosterone is pathological.

Even though most doctors will treat you with testosterone if your tests show that you are truly hypogonadal, it is still a good idea to find an anti-aging physician who understands how to treat all of your hormone imbalances, even if they are only mild or moderate.   Why wait until a condition gets so bad that your health has already deteriorated severely?

If a man gets testosterone, his libido will increase. It is important that his mate has an interest in sex that matches his.

You may want to find the same physician to treat both you and your wife. If your wife is hormone-deficient, it's not as easy for her to get a prescription to correct her hormones with bioidentical hormones as she ages. The standard of care is to NOT prescribe bioidenticals to women, but to prescribe pharmaceutical drugs to treat the symptoms of menopause.

Many women have been told by their doctors that all estrogen supplementation is harmful. These doctors do not understand the difference between dangerous horse estrogen (Premarin) and bioidentical estrogen that exactly matches the estrogen made in the human female body.   These doctors remain fearful of all hormone replacement therapy and refuse to offer it to hormonally-deficient women.

When menopausal women begin to take bioidentical estradiol (E2), their interest in sex heightens.[148] Estradiol is also known as E2. It is the estrogen made in a woman's reproductive years. Low doses of estradiol have minimal effect.[149] But higher doses of estradiol do heighten sexual interest.

Suddenly, her partner becomes VERY attractive.[150] She will report that she is enjoying sex more, is more satisfied with the frequency of sex, and is happier about her interest in sex. Additional testosterone may enhance the effect.[151] [152]

Another powerful hormone that will help the female libido is DHEA.[153] DHEA also controls thickness of the skin. A woman who has high DHEA levels will want to have sex frequently and will have youthful skin.

Look for a physician who is well-trained with lots of clinical experience. Some physicians will prescribe anything that you ask for. But that does not mean that they are knowledgeable about what they are prescribing and that they can properly manage the hormone problems.

Ask about the physician's training and the types of hormones that they frequently prescribe. The physician that you are looking for has a firm grasp of how all of the endocrine systems interact.

Best of all is a physician who has completed a fellowship in anti-aging medicine from the American Academy of Anti-Aging Medicine (A4M). Go to: http://www.a4m.com/directory.html

Doctors in alternative medicine are often excellent choices when looking for a physician. Functional medicine is one system of alternative medicine. Functional physicians train through ACAM, the American College for Advancement in Medicine.   The major state-of-the-art medical testing laboratories like Genova, Diagnos-Techs, and Doctors' Data keep physician referral lists, as well.

When your physician prescribes a hormone, he has found a deficiency of that hormone. Your physician is treating a deficiency disease, not just randomly prescribing something that might make you feel better.

Sometimes it may be a tough call for your doctor to make.   The symptoms that you report may differ from the results of your lab tests.

When this happens, the wisest physicians usually treat based on clinical findings (your symptoms and physical exam). If your physician refuses to treat you because lab tests don't prove that a deficiency exists, but you are experiencing symptoms of a hormone deficiency, you may want to get a second opinion.

Anti-aging physicians diagnose and treat mild and moderate hormone deficiency, because it preserves health. They understand that your health will deteriorate if you wait until the hormone deficiency progresses from moderate to severe deficiency. If it takes five years for a hormone deficiency to progress to a severe state, over those five years you will have poor immunity to infection, advancing atherosclerotic vascular disease, depression, obesity, and all the other problems caused by deficient hormones.

If a deficiency is proven to exist, it is ultimately your decision about what to do about it. You have a choice about whether or not to replace deficient hormones. If you decide to replace deficient hormones, there are many choices for you to make about the methods that you want to use. Use this book and your doctor's advice to help you make an informed decision.

Intelligent hormone replacement for men is an art. The goal is to bring each hormone precisely into balance with all of the others. The wise physician looks at the big picture, continually changing dosages up and down until balance is achieved. The wise physician knows how one hormone affects the other hormones. This wise physician listens to the patient and does not ignore what the patient is saying about how he feels (clinical symptoms). This is why it is important to find an experienced clinician who will listen to you and treat your individual needs.

Questions your doctor should ask:

- Do you have any prostate symptoms?
- Tighter urinary stream with age?
- Residual fluid in bladder after urination?
- Do you wake more than once to urinate at night?
- Has your P.S.A. been rising?
- When was your last prostate exam, and what were the results?
- Is fertility important, and are there fertility problems?

- Do you have a morning erection (a chubby)?
- How is your libido?
- Do you have symptoms of erectile dysfunction?
- Have you experienced decreased muscle mass and strength?
- When was your last bone density test?

Your doctor should also discuss all of the side effects of testosterone replacement, if it is needed. If your labs show suboptimal testosterone, you should be asked if you want to maintain testicular volume and sperm count.

If you do, your doctor should determine if your FSH and LH are elevated. If they are, then hCG probably won't work. If they aren't elevated, you may want to consider hCG. Or you may want to use a combination of hCG and testosterone, using hCG one or two days a week in combination with the testosterone cream or the cypionate injections. Or you may choose to use only the testosterone gels or cypionate injections.

Your doctor will want to measure DHT and estrogen if you have any prostate symptoms. Most men should probably take saw palmetto and other prostate supplements. If your progesterone is low, consider taking progesterone. It should help you to sleep better.

Follow up is done after treatment is initiated. Are any hormones too high or too low? Your doctor should ask you how you are feeling. Are you experiencing side effects? Are you feeling better? If you are using cream and you are not feeling better, maybe it isn't working for you. Check for side effects of testosterone—elevated red blood cells, elevated estrogen, elevated DHT. If you have elevated red blood cells, you may need to donate blood or just throw it away if you are not a suitable donor. If estradiol is too high, lower it with nutritional changes, and then use aromatase inhibitors. Lose fat. Check to see if PSA is increasing (PSA velocity)?

When you look for a doctor, look for a caring person with a warm heart and integrity. Avoid doctors whose only concern is to maximize profits for their HMO. Sidestep also the greedy ones, who maximize profits for themselves. Beware of any who feel that they are superior to you, "the patient," or those who are simply lazy or incompetent.

It is important that your doctor treats you as a whole person and not just a disease or set of symptoms, or worse, a checkbook. Your goal is to find a physician whose motivation comes from the heart, works hard to be of service to you, who will approach you as a unique person, and will travel with you on your quest for health.

ABOUT THE AUTHORS

J.M. Swartz M.D. and Y. L. Wright M.A. teach people about bioidentical hormones and anti-aging medicine. Dr. Swartz has a long history of training and clinical experience. Dr. Swartz received his medical degree from Baylor College of Medicine, completed an internship at Presbyterian Medical Center in San Francisco, CA., and completed a UCLA-affiliated family practice residency. Dr. Swartz also trained extensively in structural medicine in order to help patients to recover from severe chronic pain. He has served as a family practitioner for over forty years.

J.M. Swartz M.D. specializes in hormones, aging, pain, and difficult medical problems. In order to help people to recover from their medical problems, Dr. Joe has found that it is absolutely critical to balance their hormones.

Y.L. Wright M.A. focused her graduate studies on Human Anatomy and Physiology and later became proficient in many manual medicine therapies. Y.L. (Yvonne) assisted Dr. Joe (her husband) in his medical practice treating many patients labeled as "hopeless" by other medical professionals who had seen them. After working with Dr. Joe and Yvonne, most were finally able to recover from debilitating chronic pain and illnesses.

Dr. Joe and Yvonne both study with the American Academy of Anti-Aging Medicine (A4M) and review the latest research articles in the major medical journals. Because very few physicians understand the value of using bioidentical hormones or how to use them effectively, Dr. Joe and Yvonne have written the "Bioidentical Hormones" series of books in order to educate both patients and physicians about optimizing their hormones at every stage of life, no matter how young or old they are.

Dr. Joe believes that everyone has the right to receive treatment to optimize their hormones, no matter how severe the hormonal imbalance may be. When he is not seeing patients, he enjoys playing tennis, lifting weights, organic gardening, and wood-working.

REFERENCES

[1] Jäger T, Kramer J, Bätz O, Rübben H, von Ostau C, Szarvas T. [Testosterone deficiency - an underestimated risk for men? Prevalence of hypogonadism]. *Urologe A. 2013 Dec;52(12):1684-9.*

[2] Dwyer AA. Lifestyle modification can reverse hypogonadism in men with impaired glucose tolerance in the Diabetes Prevention Program. *[Abstract OR28-3]. Presented at ENDO 2012 (The Endocrine Society), June 27, 2012.*

[3] Wright YL, Swartz, JM. *Secrets About the HCG Diet! Treatment Guide, Controversy, Benefits, Risks, Side Effects, and Contraindications.* Lulu.com. 2012.

[4] Wright YL, Swartz, JM. *Secrets to Lose Toxic Belly Fat! Heal Your Sick Metabolism Using State-Of-The-Art Medical Testing and Treatment With Detoxification, Diet, Lifestyle, Supplements, and Bioidentical Hormones.* Lulu.com. 2012.

[5] Swartz JM M.D. and Wright YL M.A. *Keto Smart!: Heal Your Brain and Body With the Ten-Step Action Plan Scientifically Proven to Prevent or Reverse Obesity, Memory Loss, Alzheimer's, Diabetes, Autoimmunity, Cancer, and Heart Disease.* Lulu.com. 2019.

[6] Swartz JM M.D. and Wright YL M.A. *Secrets About Growth Hormone To Build Muscle Mass, Increase Bone Density, And Burn Body Fat!* Lulu.com 2011.

[7] Swartz JM M.D. and Wright YL M.A. *TOXIC TEETH: How a Biological (Holistic) Dentist Can Help You Cure Cancer, Facial Pain, Autoimmune, Heart, and Other Disease Caused By Infected Gums, Root Canals, Jawbone Cavitations, and Toxic Metals.* Lulu.com 2016.

[8] Carcaillon L, Brailly-Tabard S, Ancelin ML, Tzourio C, Foubert-Samier A, Dartigues JF, Guiochon-Mantel A, Scarabin PY. Low testosterone and the risk of dementia in elderly men: Impact of age and education. *Alzheimers Dement. 2013 Sep10.*

[9] Pikwer M, Giwercman A, Bergström U, Nilsson JÅ, Jacobsson LT, Turesson C. Association between testosterone levels and risk of future rheumatoid arthritis in men: a population-based case-control study. *Ann Rheum Dis. 2014 Mar;73(3):573-9.*

[10] Esser N, Legrand-Poels S, Piette J, Scheen AJ, Paquot N. Inflammation as a link between obesity, metabolic syndrome and type 2 diabetes. *Diabetes Res Clin Pract. 2014 Apr 13. pii: S0168-8227(14)00187-9.*

[11] Irwig MS. Male hypogonadism and skeletal health. Curr Opin Endocrinol Diabetes Obes. 2013 Dec;20(6):517-22.

[12] Murillo-Cuesta S, Rodríguez-de la Rosa L, Cediel R, Lassaletta L, Varela-Nieto I. The role of insulin-like growth factor-I in the physiopathology of hearing. *Front Mol Neurosci. 2011 Jul 25;4:11.*

[13] Lambooij AC, van Wely KH, Lindenbergh-Kortleve DJ, Kuijpers RW, Kliffen M, Mooy CM. Insulin-like growth factor-I and its receptor in neurovascular age-related macular degeneration. *Invest Ophthalmol Vis Sci. 2003 May;44(5):2192-8.*

[14] Tamer C, Oksuz H, Söğüt S. Serum dehydroepiandrosterone sulphate level in age-related macular degeneration. *Am J Ophthalmol. 2007 Feb;143(2):212-216.*

[15] Güder G, Allolio B, Angermann CE, Störk S. Androgen deficiency in heart failure. *Curr Heart Fail Rep. 2011 Jun;8(2):131-9.*

[16] Vignozzi L, Cellai I, Santi R, Lombardelli L, Morelli A, Comeglio P, Filippi S, Logiodice F, Carini M, Nesi G, Gacci M, Piccinni MP, Adorini L, Maggi M. Antiinflammatory effect of androgen receptor activation in human benign prostatic hyperplasia cells. *J Endocrinol. 2012 Jul;214(1):31-43.*

[17] Su JJ, Park SK, Hsieh TM. The Effect of Testosterone on Cardiovascular Disease: A Critical Review of the Literature. *Am J Mens Health. 2014 Feb 20.*

[18] Laughlin GA, Barrett-Connor E, Bergstrom J. Low serum testosterone and mortality in older men. *J Clin Endocrinol Metab. 2008 Jan;93(1):68-75*

[19] Khaw K., et al. Endogenous Testosterone and Mortality Due to All Causes, Cardiovascular Disease, and Cancer in Men. *Circulation. 2007;116:2694-2701.*

[20] Vikan T, Schirmer H, Njølstad I, Svartberg J. Endogenous sex hormones and the prospective association with cardiovascular disease and mortality in men: the Tromsø Study. *Eur J Endocrinol.* 2009 Sep;161(3):435-42.

[21] Shores MM, Matsumoto AM, Sloan KL, Kivlahan DR. Low serum testosterone and mortality in male veterans. *Arch Intern Med.* 2006 Aug 14;166(15):1660-5.

[22] Khaw KT, Dowsett M, Folkerd E, Bingham S, Wareham N, Luben R, Welch A, Day N. Endogenous testosterone and mortality due to all causes, cardiovascular disease, and cancer in men: European prospective investigation into cancer in Norfolk(EPIC-Norfolk) Prospective Population Study. *Circulation.* 2007 Dec 4;116(23):2694-701.

[23] Hoffman MA, DeWolf WC, Morgentaler A. Is low serum free testosterone a marker for high grade prostate cancer? *J Urol.* 2000 Mar;163(3):824-7.

[24] Morgentaler A. Rapidly shifting concepts regarding androgens and prostate cancer. *Scientific World Journal.* 2009 Jul 27;9:685-90.

[25] Cintron JR, Asadi FK, Malakouti S, Abcarian HA. Androgen induces ornithine decarboxylase gene expression in colonic cell line HT-29. *Dis Colon Rectum.* 1996 Apr;39(4):406-9.

[26] Pike CJ, Rosario ER, Nguyen TV. Androgens, aging, and Alzheimer's disease. *Endocrine.* 2006 Apr;29(2):233-41. Review.

[27] Chu LW, Tam S, Lee PW, Wong RL, Yik PY, Tsui W, Song Y, Cheung BM, Morley JE, Lam KS. Bioavailable testosterone is associated with a reduced risk of amnestic mild cognitive impairment in older men. *Clin Endocrinol (Oxf).* 2008Apr;68(4):589-98.

[28] Kapoor D, Jones TH. Androgen deficiency as a predictor of metabolic syndrome in aging men: an opportunity for intervention? *Drugs Aging.* 2008;25(5):357-69. Review.

[29] Tsilidis KK, Rohrmann S, McGlynn KA, Nyante SJ, Lopez DS, Bradwin G, Feinleib M, Joshu CE, Kanarek N, Nelson WG, Selvin E, Platz EA. Association between endogenous sex steroid hormones and inflammatory biomarkers in US men. *Andrology.* 2013 Nov;1(6):919-28.

[30] Boddi V, Barbaro V, McNieven P, Maggi M, Rotella CM. Present and future association between obesity and hypogonadism in Italian male. *Arch Ital Urol Androl.* 2014 Mar 28;86(1):26-32.

[31] De Pergola G. The adipose tissue metabolism: role of testosterone and dehydroepiandrosterone. *Int J Obes Relat Metab Disord.* 2000 Jun;24 Suppl2:S59-63. Review.

[32] Korenman SG, Morley JE, Mooradian AD, Davis SS, Kaiser FE, Silver AJ, Viosca SP, Garza D. Secondary hypogonadism in older men: its relation to impotence. *J Clin Endocrinol Metab.* 1990 Oct;71(4):963-9.

[33] Khaw K., et al. Endogenous Testosterone and Mortality Due to All Causes, Cardiovascular Disease, and Cancer in Men. *Circulation.* 2007;116:2694-2701.

[34] Hogervorst E, Bandelow S, Moffat SD. Increasing testosterone levels and effects on cognitive functions in elderly men and women: a review. *Curr Drug Targets CNS Neurol Disord.* 2005 Oct;4(5):531-40. Review.

[35] Travison TG, Araujo AB, O'Donnell AB, Kupelian V, McKinlay JB. A population-level decline in serum testosterone levels in American men. *J Clin Endocrinol Metab.* 2007 Jan;92(1):196-202.

[36] Perheentupa A, Mäkinen J, Laatikainen T, Vierula M, Skakkebaek NE, Andersson AM, Toppari J. A cohort effect on serum testosterone levels in Finnish men. *Eur J Endocrinol.* 2013 Jan 17;168(2):227-33.

[37] Nahoul K, Roger M. Age-related decline of plasma bioavailable testosterone in adult men. *J Steroid Biochem.* 1990 Feb;35(2):293-9.

[38] Bonde JP. Male reproductive organs are at risk from environmental hazards. *Asian J Androl.* 2010 Mar;12(2):152-6. Review.

[39] Cumming DC, Quigley ME, Yen SS. Acute suppression of circulating testosterone levels by cortisol in men. *J Clin Endocrinol Metab.* 1983 Sep;57(3):671-3.

40 Coward RM, Rajanahally S, Kovac JR, Smith RP, Pastuszak AW, Lipshultz LI. Anabolic steroid induced hypogonadism in young men. *J Urol.* 2013 Dec;190(6):2200-5.

41 Lašaitė L, Ceponis J, Preikša RT, Zilaitienė B. Impaired emotional state, quality of life and cognitive functions in young hypogonadal men. *Andrologia.* 2013 Dec 8.

42 Tweed JO, Hsia SH, Lutfy K, Friedman TC. The endocrine effects of nicotine and cigarette smoke. *Trends Endocrinol Metab.* 2012 Jul;23(7):334-42.

43 Merza Z. Chronic use of opioids and the endocrine system. *Horm Metab Res.* 2010 Aug;42(9):621-6.

44 Van Thiel DH, Gavaler JS, Eagon PK, Chiao YB, Cobb CF, Lester R. Alcohol and sexual function. *Pharmacol Biochem Behav.* 1980;13 Suppl 1:125-9. Review.

45 Tsujimura A, Takao T, Miyagawa Y, Okuyama A. [Bone and Men's Health. Testosterone and lifestyle disease]. *Clin Calcium.* 2010 Feb;20(2):217-23. Japanese.

46 Mendiola J, Jørgensen N, Andersson AM, Calafat AM, Ye X, Redmon JB, Drobnis EZ, Wang C, Sparks A, Thurston SW, Liu F, Swan SH. Are environmental levels of bisphenol a associated with reproductive function in fertile men? *Environ Health Perspect.* 2010 Sep;118(9):1286-91

47 Bain J. Testosterone and the aging male: to treat or not to treat? *Maturitas.* 2010 May;66(1):16-22.

48 Castelo-Branco C, Cancelo MJ, Villero J, Nohales F, Juliá MD. Management of post-menopausal vaginal atrophy and atrophic vaginitis. *Maturitas.* 2005 Nov 15;52 Suppl 1:S46-52.

49 Magon N, Chauhan M, Malik S, Shah D. Sexuality in midlife: Where the passion goes? *J Midlife Health.* 2012 Jul;3(2):61-5.

50 Schulman C, Lunenfeld B. The ageing male. *World J Urol.* 2002 May;20(1):4-10. Review.

51 Nappi RE, Lachowsky M. Menopause and sexuality: prevalence of symptoms and impact on quality of life. *Maturitas.* 2009 Jun 20;63(2):138-41.

52 Freeman EW, Sammel MD, Lin H, Nelson DB. Associations of hormones and menopausal status with depressed mood in women with no history of depression. *Arch Gen Psychiatry.* 2006 Apr;63(4):375-82.

53 Graziottin A, Leiblum SR. Biological and psychosocial pathophysiology of female sexual dysfunction during the menopausal transition. *J Sex Med.* 2005 Sep;2 Suppl 3:133-45. Review.

54 Heller CG, M.D., Ph.D. and Myers G, M.D. The male climacteric, its symptomatology, diagnosis and treatment. *Journal of the American Medical Association* 1944; 126(8):472-477.

55 Dwyer AA. Lifestyle modification can reverse hypogonadism in men with impaired glucose tolerance in the Diabetes Prevention Program. *[Abstract OR28-3]. Presented at ENDO 2012 (The Endocrine Society), June 27, 2012.*

56 Shibata Y, Ito K, Suzuki K, Nakano K, et al. Changes in the endocrine environment of the human prostate transition zone with aging: simultaneous quantitative analysis of prostatic sex steroids and comparison with human prostatic histological composition. *Prostate.* 2000 Jan;42(1):45-55.

57 Williams G. Aromatase up-regulation, insulin and raised intracellular oestrogens in men, induce adiposity, metabolic syndrome and prostate disease, via aberrant ER-α and GPER signalling. *Mol Cell Endocrinol.* 2012 Apr 4;351(2):269-78.

58 Fuhrman BJ, Schairer C, Gail MH, Boyd-Morin J, Xu X, Sue LY, Buys SS, Isaacs C, Keefer LK, Veenstra TD, Berg CD, Hoover RN, Ziegler RG. Estrogen metabolism and risk of breast cancer in postmenopausal women. *J Natl Cancer Inst.* 2012 Feb 22;104(4):326-39.

59 Bosland MC. Sex steroids and prostate carcinogenesis: integrated, multifactorial working hypothesis. *Ann N Y Acad Sci.* 2006 Nov;1089:168-76.

60 Yu S, Zhang Y, Yuen MT, Zou C, Danielpour D, Chan FL. 17-Beta-estradiol induces neoplastic transformation in prostatic epithelial cells. *Cancer Lett.* 2011 May 1;304(1):8-20.

61 Morgentaler A, Traish AM. Shifting the paradigm of testosterone and prostate cancer: the saturation model and the limits of androgen-dependent growth. *Eur Urol.* 2009 Feb;55(2):310-20.

62 Colmou A. [Estrogens and vascular thrombosis]. Soins Gynecol Obstet Pueric Pediatr. 1982

Sep;(16):39-41. French.

[63] Abbott RD, Launer LJ, Rodriguez BL, Ross GW, Wilson PW, Masaki KH, Strozyk D, Curb JD, Yano K, Popper JS, Petrovitch H. Serum estradiol and risk of stroke in elderly men. *Neurology.* 2007 Feb 20;68(8):563-8.

[64] Tyler CR, Spary C, Gibson R, Santos EM, Shears J, Hill EM. Accounting for differences in estrogenic responses in rainbow trout (Oncorhynchus mykiss: Salmonidae) and roach (Rutilus rutilus: Cyprinidae) exposed to effluents from wastewater treatment works. *Environ Sci Technol.* 2005 Apr 15;39(8):2599-607.

[65] Wright YL, Swartz, JM. *Secrets to Lose Toxic Belly Fat! Heal Your Sick Metabolism Using State-Of-The-Art Medical Testing and Treatment With Detoxification, Diet, Lifestyle, Supplements, and Bioidentical Hormones.* Lulu.com. 2012.

[66] Swartz JM M.D. and Wright YL M.A. *Keto Smart!: Heal Your Brain and Body With the Ten-Step Action Plan Scientifically Proven to Prevent or Reverse Obesity, Memory Loss, Alzheimer's, Diabetes, Autoimmunity, Cancer, and Heart Disease.* Lulu.com. 2019.

[67] Wright YL, Swartz, JM. Secrets to Lose Toxic Belly Fat! Heal Your Sick Metabolism Using State-Of-The-Art Medical Testing and Treatment With Detoxification, Diet, Lifestyle, Supplements, and Bioidentical Hormones. Lulu.com. 2012.

[68] Wright YL, Swartz, JM. Secrets about Growth Hormone to Build Muscle Mass, Increase Bone Density, and Burn Body Fat! Lulu.com. 2012.

[69] Kuzma M, Homerova Z, Dlesk A, Koller T, Killinger Z, Vanuga P, Lazurova I, Tomkova S, Payer J. Effect of growth hormone on bone status in growth hormone-deficient adults. *Bratisl Lek Listy.* 2013;114(12):689-95.

[70] Muniyappa R, Sorkin JD, Veldhuis JD, Harman SM, Münzer T, Bhasin S, Blackman MR. Long-term testosterone supplementation augments overnight growth hormone secretion in healthy older men. *Am J Physiol Endocrinol Metab.* 2007 Sep;293(3):E769-75.

[71] Rosén T, Edén S, Larson G, Wilhelmsen L, Bengtsson BA. Cardiovascular risk factors in adult patients with growth hormone deficiency. *Acta Endocrinol (Copenh).* 1993 Sep;129(3):195-200.

[72] Van Cauter E, Leproult R, Plat L. Age-related changes in slow wave sleep and REM sleep and relationship with growth hormone and cortisol levels in healthy men. *JAMA.* 2000 Aug 16;284(7):861-8.

[73] Perls TT, Reisman NR, Olshansky SJ. Provision or distribution of growth hormone for "antiaging": clinical and legal issues. *JAMA.* 2005 Oct 26;294(16):2086-90.

[74] Jenkins PJ, Mukherjee A, Shalet SM. Does growth hormone cause cancer? *Clin Endocrinol (Oxf).* 2006 Feb;64(2):115-21. Review.

[75] Roddam AW, et al. Insulin-like growth factors, their binding proteins, and prostate cancer risk: analysis of individual patient data from 12 prospective studies. *Ann Intern Med.* 2008 Oct 7;149(7):461-71, W83-8.

[76] Lulu C, Pin L, Yan L. The effect of different nutritional states on puberty onset and the expression of hypothalamic Kiss1/kisspepetin. *J Pediatr Endocrinol Metab.* 2013;26(1-2):61-9.

[77] Jasik CB, Lustig RH. Adolescent obesity and puberty: the "perfect storm". *Ann N Y Acad Sci.* 2008;1135:265-79.

[78] Wagner IV, Sergeyev E, Dittrich K, Gesing J, Neef M, Adler M, Geserick M,Pfäffle RW, Körner A, Kiess W. [Does childhood obesity affect sexual development?]. *Bundesgesundheitsblatt Gesundheitsforschung Gesundheitsschutz.*2013 Apr;56(4):504-10.

[79] Dwyer AA. Lifestyle modification can reverse hypogonadism in men with impaired glucose tolerance in the Diabetes Prevention Program. [Abstract OR28-3]. *Presented at ENDO 2012 (The Endocrine Society), June 27, 2012.*

[80] Wright YL, Swartz, JM. Secrets to Lose Toxic Belly Fat! Heal Your Sick Metabolism Using State-Of-

The-Art Medical Testing and Treatment With Detoxification, Diet, Lifestyle, Supplements, and Bioidentical Hormones. Lulu.com. 2012.

[81] American College of Sports Medicine Position Stand. The recommended quantity and quality of exercise for developing and maintaining cardiorespiratory and muscular fitness, and flexibility in healthy adults. *Med Sci Sports Exerc. 1998 Jun;30(6):975-91. Review.*

[82] Schöpper H, Palme R, Ruf T, Huber S. Chronic stress in pregnant guinea pigs (Cavia aperea f. porcellus) attenuates long-term stress hormone levels and body weight gain, but not reproductive output. *J Comp Physiol B. 2011 Jun 7.*

[83] Santeusanio F, Di Loreto C, Lucidi P, Murdolo G, De Cicco A, Parlanti N, Piccioni F, De Feo P. Diabetes and exercise. *J Endocrinol Invest. 2003 Sep;26(9):937-40. Review.*

[84] Hopps E, Caimi G. Exercise in obesity management. *J Sports Med Phys Fitness. 2011 Jun;51(2):275-82.*

[85] Bodenant M, Kuulasmaa K, Wagner A, Kee F, Palmieri L, Ferrario MM, Montaye M, Amouyel P, Dallongeville J; for the MORGAM Project. Measures of Abdominal Adiposity and the Risk of Stroke: The Monica Risk, Genetics, Archiving and Monograph (MORGAM) Study. *Stroke. 2011 Oct;42(10):2872-2877.*

[86] Wright YL, Swartz, JM. Secrets to Lose Toxic Belly Fat! Heal Your Sick Metabolism Using State-Of-The-Art Medical Testing and Treatment With Detoxification, Diet, Lifestyle, Supplements, and Bioidentical Hormones. Lulu.com. 2012.

[87] Gerson M. The cure of advanced cancer by diet therapy: a summary of 30 years of clinical experimentation. *Physiol Chem Phys. 1978;10(5):449-64.*

[88] Uchikawa T, Yasutake A, Kumamoto Y, Maruyama I, Kumamoto S, Ando Y. The influence of Parachlorella beyerinckii CK-5 on the absorption and excretion of methylmercury (MeHg) in mice. *J Toxicol Sci. 2010;35(1):101-5.*

[89] Pore RS. Detoxification of chlordecone poisoned rats with chlorella and chlorella derived sporopollenin. *Drug Chem Toxicol. 1984;7(1):57-71.*

[90] Huang Z, Li L, Huang G, Yan Q, Shi B, Xu X. Growth-inhibitory and metal-binding proteins in Chlorella vulgaris exposed to cadmium or zinc. *Aquat Toxicol. 2009 Jan 18;91(1):54-61.*

[91] Wright YL, Swartz, JM. Secrets to Lose Toxic Belly Fat! Heal Your Sick Metabolism Using State-Of-The-Art Medical Testing and Treatment With Detoxification, Diet, Lifestyle, Supplements, and Bioidentical Hormones. Lulu.com. 2012.

[92] Hoyos CM, Killick R, Yee BJ, Grunstein RR, Liu PY. Effects of testosterone therapy on sleep and breathing in obese men with severe obstructive sleep apnoea: a randomized placebo-controlled trial. *Clin Endocrinol (Oxf). 2012Oct;77(4):599-607.*

[93] Drager LF, Polotsky VY, Lorenzi-Filho G. Obstructive sleep apnea: an emerging risk factor for atherosclerosis. *Chest. 2011 Aug;140(2):534-42.*

[94] Calof OM, Singh AB, Lee ML, et al. Adverse events associated with testosterone replacement in middle-aged and older men: a meta-analysis of randomized, placebo-controlled trials. *The Journals of Gerontology A. 2005;60(11):1451–1457.*

[95] Ismailogullari S, Korkmaz C, Peker Y, Bayram F, Karaca Z, Aksu M. Impact of long-term gonadotropin replacement treatment on sleep in men with idiopathic hypogonadotropic hypogonadism. *The Journal of Sexual Medicine. 2011;8(7):2090–2097.*

[96] Bhasin S, Cunningham GR, Hayes FJ, et al. Testosterone therapy in men with androgen deficiency syndromes: an endocrine society clinical practice guideline. *The Journal of Clinical Endocrinology & Metabolism. 2010;95(6):2536–2559.*

[97] Calof OM, Singh AB, Lee ML, et al. Adverse events associated with testosterone replacement in middle-aged and older men: a meta-analysis of randomized, placebo-controlled trials. *The Journals of Gerontology A. 2005;60(11):1451–1457.*

[98] Hanafy HM. Testosterone therapy and obstructive sleep apnea: is there a real connection? *The Journal of Sexual Medicine. 2007;4(5):1241–1246.*

[99] Curran MJ, Bihrle W., III Dramatic rise in prostate-specific antigen after androgen replacement in a hypogonadal man with occult adenocarcinoma of the prostate. *Urology. 1999;53(2):423–424.*

[100] Rhoden EL, Morgentaler A. Risks of testosterone-replacement therapy and recommendations for monitoring. *The New England Journal of Medicine. 2004;350(5):482–492.*

[101] Sengupta S, Duncan HJ, Macgregor RJ, Russell JM. The development of prostate cancer despite late onset androgen deficiency. *International Journal of Urology. 2005;12(9):847–848.*

[102] Yassin AA, Saad F. Improvement of sexual function in Men with late-onset hypogonadism treated with testosterone only. *The Journal of Sexual Medicine. 2007;4(2):497–501.*

[103] Yassin AA, Saad F. Testosterone and erectile dysfunction. *Journal of Andrology. 2008;29(6):593–604.*

[104] Coward RM, Simhan J, Carson CC. Prostate-specific antigen changes and prostate cancer in hypogonadal men treated with testosterone replacement therapy. *BJU International. 2009;103(9):1179–1183.*

[105] Morgentaler A. Testosterone replacement therapy and prostate cancer. *Urologic Clinics of North America. 2007;34(4):555–563.*

[106] Calof OM, Singh AB, Lee ML, et al. Adverse events associated with testosterone replacement in middle-aged and older men: a meta-analysis of randomized, placebo-controlled trials. *The Journals of Gerontology A. 2005;60(11):1451–1457.*

[107] Kaufman JM, Graydon RJ. Androgen replacement after curative radical prostatectomy for prostate cancer in hypogonadal men. *The Journal of Urology. 2004;172(3):920–922.*

[108] Agarwal PK, Oefelein MG. Testosterone replacement therapy after primary treatment for prostate cancer. *The Journal of Urology. 2005;173(2):533–536.*

[109] Sarosdy MF. Testosterone replacement for hypogonadism after treatment of early prostate cancer with brachytherapy. *Cancer. 2007;109(3):536–541.*

[110] Glueck CJ, Wang P. Testosterone therapy, thrombosis, thrombophilia, cardiovascular events. *Metabolism. 2014 Aug;63(8):989-94.*

[111] Camacho EM, Huhtaniemi IT, O'Neill TW, Finn JD, Pye SR, Lee DM, Tajar A, Bartfai G, Boonen S, Casanueva FF, Forti G, Giwercman A, Han TS, Kula K, KeevilB, Lean ME, Pendleton N, Punab M, Vanderschueren D, Wu FC; EMAS Group. Age-associated changes in hypothalamic-pituitary-testicular function in middle-aged and older men are modified by weight change and lifestyle factors: longitudinal results from the European Male Ageing Study. *Eur J Endocrinol. 2013 Feb 20;168(3):445-55.*

[112] Adimoelja A. Phytochemicals and the breakthrough of traditional herbs in the management of sexual dysfunctions. *Int J Androl. 2000;23 Suppl 2:82-4.*

[113] Yin XX, Chen ZQ, Liu ZJ, Ma QJ, Dang GT. Icariine stimulates proliferation and differentiation of human osteoblasts by increasing production of bone morphogenetic protein 2. *Chin Med J (Engl). 2007 Feb 5;120(3):204-10.*

[114] Yakubu MT, Afolayan AJ. Anabolic and androgenic activities of Bulbine natalensis stem in male Wistar rats. *Pharm Biol. 2010 May;48(5):568-76.*

[115] Yakubu MT, Afolayan AJ. Reproductive toxicologic evaluations of Bulbine natalensis Baker stem extract in albino rats. *Theriogenology. 2009 Aug;72(3):322-32.*

[116] Yakubu MT, Afolayan AJ. Effect of aqueous extract of Bulbine natalensis(Baker) stem on the sexual behaviour of male rats. *Int J Androl. 2009 Dec;32(6):629-36.*

[117] Shukla KK, Mahdi AA, Ahmad MK, Shankhwar SN, Rajender S, Jaiswar SP. Mucuna pruriens improves male fertility by its action on the hypothalamus-pituitary-gonadal axis. *Fertil Steril. 2009 Dec;92(6):1934-40.*

[118] Katzenschlager R, Evans A, Manson A, Patsalos PN, Ratnaraj N, Watt H, Timmermann L, Van der

Giessen R, Lees AJ. Mucuna pruriens in Parkinson's disease:a double blind clinical and pharmacological study. *J Neurol Neurosurg Psychiatry. 2004 Dec;75(12):1672-7.*

[119] Tambi MI, Imran MK, Henkel RR. Standardised water-soluble extract of Eurycoma longifolia, Tongkat ali, as testosterone booster for managing men with late-onset hypogonadism? *Andrologia. 2012 May;44 Suppl 1:226-30.*

[120] Taylor, L. The Healing Power of Rainforest Herbs: A Guide to Understanding and Using Herbal Medicinals. *Square One Publishers, 2005.*

[121] Gonzales GF, Miranda S, Nieto J, Fernández G, Yucra S, Rubio J, Yi P, Gasco M. Red maca (Lepidium meyenii) reduced prostate size in rats. *Reprod Biol Endocrinol. 2005 Jan 20;3:5.*

[122] Malviya N, Jain S, Gupta VB, Vyas S. Recent studies on aphrodisiac herbs for the management of male sexual dysfunction--a review. *Acta Pol Pharm. 2011 Jan-Feb;68(1):3-8. Review.*

[123] Saarinen N, Joshi SC, Ahotupa M, Li X, Ammälä J, Mäkelä S, Santti R. No evidence for the in vivo activity of aromatase-inhibiting flavonoids. *J Steroid Biochem Mol Biol. 2001 Sep;78(3):231-9.*

[124] Waynsberg J. Aphrodisiacs: Contribution to the clinical validation of the traditional use of Ptychopetalum guyanna. *Presented at the First International Congress on Ethnopharmacology, Strasbourg, France, June 5-9, 1990.*

[125] Sternbach H. Age-associated testosterone decline in men: clinical issues for psychiatry. *Am J Psychiatry. 1998 Oct;155(10):1310-8.*

[126] http://www.nlm.nih.gov/medlineplus/druginfo/natural/759.html

[127] Adeniyi AA, Brindley GS, Pryor JP, Ralph DJ. Yohimbine in the treatment of orgasmic dysfunction. *Asian J Androl. 2007 May;9(3):403-7.*

[128] Sohn, M, Sikora, R. Ginkgo biloba extract in the therapy of erectile dysfunction. *Journal of Sex Education & Therapy, Vol 17(1), 1991, 53-61.*

[129] Cohen AJ, Bartlik B. Ginkgo biloba for antidepressant-induced sexual dysfunction. *J Sex Marital Ther. 1998 Apr-Jun;24(2):139-43.*

[130] Wilborn C, Taylor L, Poole C, Foster C, Willoughby D, Kreider R. Effects of a purported aromatase and 5α-reductase inhibitor on hormone profiles in college-age men. *Int J Sport Nutr Exerc Metab. 2010 Dec;20(6):457-65.*

[131] Steels E, Rao A, Vitetta L. Physiological Aspects of Male Libido Enhanced by Standardized Trigonella foenum-graecum Extract and Mineral Formulation. *Phytother Res. 2011 Sep;25(9):1294-300.*

[132] Prasad AS. Clinical, immunological, anti-inflammatory and antioxidant roles of zinc. *Exp Gerontol. 2008 May;43(5):370-7. Review.*

[133] Stanislavov R, Nikolova V. Treatment of erectile dysfunction with pycnogenol and L-arginine. *J Sex Marital Ther. 2003 May-Jun;29(3):207-13.*

[134] Lebret T, Hervé JM, Gorny P, Worcel M, Botto H. Efficacy and safety of a novel combination of L-arginine glutamate and yohimbine hydrochloride: a new oral therapy for erectile dysfunction. *Eur Urol. 2002 Jun;41(6):608-13; discussion 613.*

[135] Cormio L, De Siati M, Lorusso F, Selvaggio O, Mirabella L, Sanguedolce F, Carrieri G. Oral L-citrulline supplementation improves erection hardness in men with mild erectile dysfunction. *Urology. 2011 Jan;77(1):119-22.*

[136] Naghii MR, Mofid M, Asgari AR, Hedayati M, Daneshpour MS. Comparative effects of daily and weekly boron supplementation on plasma steroid hormones and proinflammatory cytokines. *J Trace Elem Med Biol. 2011 Jan;25(1):54-8.*

[137] Angwafor F 3rd, Anderson ML. An open label, dose response study to determine the effect of a dietary supplement on dihydrotestosterone, testosterone and estradiol levels in healthy males. *J Int Soc Sports Nutr. 2008 Aug 12;5:12.*

[138] Anderson ML. Evaluation of Resettin® on serum hormone levels in sedentary males. *J Int Soc Sports Nutr. 2014 Aug 23;11:43.*

139 Zitzmann M, Nieschlag E. Hormone substitution in male hypogonadism. Mol Cell *Endocrinol. 2000 Mar 30;161(1-2):73-88. Review.*

140 Efficacy and safety of highly purified urinary follicle-stimulating hormone with human chorionic gonadotropin for treating men with isolated hypogonadotropic hypogonadism. *European Metrodin HP Study Group. Fertil Steril. 1998 Aug;70(2):256-62.*

141 Tsujimura A, Matsumiya K, Takao T, Miyagawa Y, Takada S, Koga M, Iwasa A, Takeyama M, Okuyama A. Treatment with human chorionic gonadotropin for PADAM: a preliminary report. *Aging Male. 2005 Sep-Dec;8(3-4):175-9.*

142 Kalinchenko Slu, Tishova IuA, Vorslov LO, Nesterov MN. [Partial androgen deficiency in aging male (Padam syndrome): terminology and current approaches to choice of replacement hormonal therapy]. *Urologiia. 2006 Nov-Dec;(6):28, 31-4.*

143 http://abcnews.go.com/Sports/nfl-star-wanted-child-faces-drug-suspension/story?id=23790350

144 Naghii MR, Mofid M, Asgari AR, Hedayati M, Daneshpour MS. Comparative effects of daily and weekly boron supplementation on plasma steroid hormones and proinflammatory cytokines. *J Trace Elem Med Biol. 2011 Jan;25(1):54-8.*

145 Henkel RR, Wang R, Bassett SH, Chen T, Liu N, Zhu Y, Tambi MI. Tongkat Ali as a potential herbal supplement for physically active male and female seniors—a pilot study. *Phytother Res. 2014 Apr;28(4):544-50.*

146 Boonen S, Vanderschueren D, Cheng XG, Verbeke G, Dequeker J, Geusens P, Broos P, Bouillon R. Age-related (type II) femoral neck osteoporosis in men: biochemical evidence for both hypovitaminosis D- and androgen deficiency-induced bone resorption. *J Bone Miner Res. 1997 Dec;12(12):2119-26.*

147 Extent and nature of testosterone use [news release]. *Fairfield, Conn: IMS Health; September 2006.*

148 Seredynski AL, Balthazart J, Christophe VJ, Ball GF, Cornil CA. Neuroestrogens rapidly regulate sexual motivation but not performance. *J Neurosci. 2013 Jan 2;33(1):164-74.*

149 Huang A, Yaffe K, Vittinghoff E, Kuppermann M, Addis I, Hanes V, Quan J, Grady D. The effect of ultralow-dose transdermal estradiol on sexual function in postmenopausal women. *Am J Obstet Gynecol. 2008 Mar;198(3):265.e1-7.*

150 Roney JR, Simmons ZL, Gray PB. Changes in estradiol predict within-women shifts in attraction to facial cues of men's testosterone. *Psychoneuroendocrinology. 2011 Jun;36(5):742-9.*

151 Flöter A, Nathorst-Böös J, Carlström K, von Schoultz B. Addition of testosterone to estrogen replacement therapy in oophorectomized women: effects on sexuality and well-being. *Climacteric. 2002 Dec;5(4):357-65.*

152 Davis SR, McCloud P, Strauss BJ, Burger H. Testosterone enhances estradiol's effects on postmenopausal bone density and sexuality. *Maturitas. 2008 Sep-Oct;61(1-2):17-26.*

153 Bloch M, Meiboom H, Zaig I, Schreiber S, Abramov L. The use of dehydroepiandrosterone in the treatment of hypoactive sexual desire disorder: A report of gender differences. *Eur Neuropsychopharmacol. 2012 Oct 17.*

www.ingramcontent.com/pod-product-compliance
Lightning Source LLC
Chambersburg PA
CBHW031232280526
45784CB00004B/1543